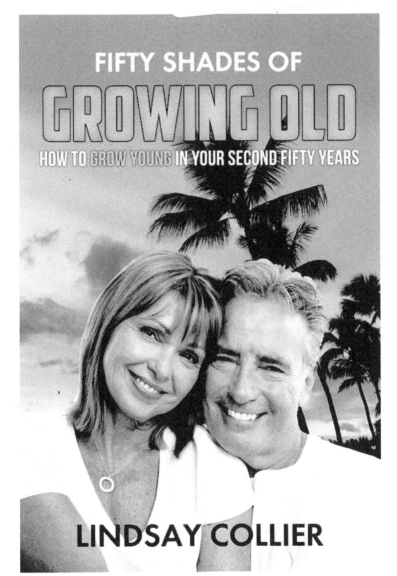

FIFTY SHADES OF
GROWING OLD
HOW TO GROW YOUNG IN YOUR SECOND FIFTY YEARS

LINDSAY COLLIER

Copyright – 2018

Lindsay Collier

**ISBN-13:
978-1725713444**

**ISBN-10:
1725713446**

Table of Contents

Introduction

It's been said that "Old age is like flying an airplane through a storm. Once you are on board there's nothing you can do." Do you believe that? I don't! That's why I wrote my book, _How To Live Happily Ever After; 12 Things You Can Do to Live Forever._ I've had some wonderful feedback from folks who were inspired by the ideas expressed in this book. And this, in turn, inspired me to begin my blog, The Growing Young Site, which is full of some very creative ideas to add zest to the lives of seniors (or anyone for that matter). If you are old enough to become a member of AARP you will find these ideas to be very valuable and exciting.

If you've been an AARP member for longer than you would like to admit, you will find some very good news here that may make you feel a lot younger. For several years I added weekly posts to _The Growing Young Site_ and, as I looked back on these, I felt it would be great to share these in book form. After all, I can't take them with me when I _buy the farm_. I have a lot of things to share on this topic, and I can't think of a better way than to continue to post on my blog, and to share this in book form with you.

I love to write, and am also an avid reader. The thoughts I will be sharing with you come from a combination of my vast (I'm not going to tell you how vast) experience and observations combined with my reading and studies. I think you will find most of them very creative, different, and exciting – and maybe a few of them will be a bit on the crazy side as well. In my past life I was an engineer and an expert in creativity and innovation at a major US corporation. After an early retirement I began my career as an author, consultant, and speaker.

I have written 12 books which take a creative look at certain aspects of life. In my **"Living Your Life to the Fullest'** series, I focus on topics that can add real zest to your life. And, in my **"Creativity, Innovation, and Change** "series I share some of the creative material I've developed and used in my earlier years focusing largely on teams and organizations. You can see all my books on my Amazon author page at amazon.com/author/lindsaycollier. They are also available as Kindle books and EBooks through Smashwords, Kobo, Barnes and Noble, and other sites.

How to read this book

My initial title was going to be, "_Scattered Thoughts on Growing Young_". This really is a book of scattered thoughts. They are short blurbs because I like 'short and to the point', and I think you do too. You can read this from cover to cover, or just open to any page and see what greets you. Keep a copy on your nightstand and read a couple of the blurbs before going to bed each night. It will give your brain some things to ponder while you sleep. And keep a copy in your bathroom for some multi-tasking. As a matter of fact, maybe you should have a copy in every room in the house (and the car, the garage, the tool shed, the attic etc.) The ideas are in no particular sequence or order of importance. Just like my **Growing Young Site** blog, I share random thoughts that come to me regarding how to stay young. I'm hoping each of these will be a fun learning experience for you. I also hope you will put these to use to add zest to your lives. They've worked for me – and I'm pretty sure they will work for you.

For each of the thoughts I have also added a quotation or two that should provide you with a little extra food for thought. There may be a bit of repetition in these posts, but many of the points well deserve repetition.

I hope you enjoy it and, if so, **please leave an honest review on the Amazon book site**. So, let's get her done!

*"Life's journey is not to
arrive at the grave safely
in a well preserved body,
but rather to skid in sideways,
totally used up and worn out, shouting Wo'hoo,
'Man, what a ride"!*

George Carlin

What If the Hokey Pokey Really Is What It's All About?

Several years ago I bought a hat with this caption on it. For some reason, when I put this hat on I tend to loosen up. This thought reminds me that perhaps I shouldn't take life so seriously. Don't take me wrong – there is definitely a serious side to living a happy life. But perhaps we can get to that point by letting go of our feeling that life is so serious

For those of you who are golfers (or perhaps engage in other similar sports) you may already have noticed that sometimes the harder you try, the worse you become. My worst days of golf are usually those times when I'm trying too hard. When that happens, I often tell myself to "loosen up". Don't be so serious and just let it flow. The results are sometimes amazing. I found this also to be true when I was an active skier and tennis player (oh to have those days back again). In my book **, How To Live Happily Ever After; 12 Things You Can Do To Live Forever**, I give an example that might just help you to change your thinking in this regard:

The nucleus accounts for almost all the atom's solidarity yet occupies one million millionth of its total volume. The rest is empty space (with electrons spinning around). Bodies are mostly empty space. The solid matter for all the human bodies on earth lumped together would be no bigger than a pea. The solid matter for the entire world would fit inside a football stadium.

Kind of puts a perspective on things, doesn't it? So the next time you find yourself being much too serious, take a good deep breath, and ask yourself. "What if the Hokey Pokey is what it's all about?" Lighten up, loosen up, and just go with the flow. You may really surprise yourself!

Speaking of lightening up, let me leave you with some sad news about the loss of the creator of the *Hokey Pokey.*

Larry LaPrise, author of 'The Hokey Pokey', dead at 93

There's sad news in the entertainment world. Larry LaPrise, who wrote the song and dance classic, 'The Hokey Pokey', is dead at 93. His funeral went off with only one hitch. While transferring Larry to his coffin, they put his left leg in, and that's when the trouble began.

"You can't help growing older. But you don't have to grow old."

Stay Young by Continually Tapping Your Creativity

I admit, I'm rather bias about the importance of creative thinking in our lives. Early on in my career as an engineer I made an observation that has stuck with me for many years. I noticed that, for the most part, people tended to leave their right brains at the gate when going to work. So I began an intensive study of the field of creative thinking and became somewhat of an expert in the area of how to use creative thinking in work and personal lives. Along the way I've made hundreds of presentations on this topic, and trained many to become creative process facilitators.

As we age, many of us lose our incentive to use our creative thinking capacity. The result is that we may lose one of the major sources of excitement and innovation in our everyday lives. Being able to continuously tap your creativity is an important part of living a happy and exciting life.

Creativity is often referred to as "thinking outside the box". Our thinking tends to be limited by what we see as the rules of possibility sometimes called "paradigms". The older we are, the more time we've had to build these paradigms into our thinking. Children are rarely limited in their thinking until their parents, teachers, and other various forms of elders have had a chance to orient them to the "rules".

Sometimes our "fear of failure" gets in the way. We won't try something new and different because we are afraid of failing, which is often considered bad. But, remember, many failures are just pathways to new opportunities. It's been said that "*everywhere you trip is an opportunity*". So maybe you need to fail quickly so you can succeed sooner. And don't worry too much about being first with an idea. As they say, "The early bird gets the worm but the second mouse gets the cheese." So for us to tap our creativity we need to "break the rules" and here are a few ways to do this. My books, ***How To Live Happily Ever After,*** and ***Organizational Mental Floss***, have a lot more techniques.

Recognize your creative capacity – Everyone (you and me included) comes loaded with an incredible capacity for creativity. The problem is that we experience things in our lives that result in a build-up of blockages. Over time these blockages erode our self-confidence so that most people begin to believe that they are just not that creative. Ask your friends and associates if they are creative and you'll find most of them will hedge a bit, or just say no.

So the first thing I want you to do is to tell yourself that **you are incredibly creative**. Go ahead – do it now. And keep telling yourself this until you really, truly believe it. And, as you convince yourself of your creative capacity don't forget to throw in the proclamation that you can really make a difference in everything in which you are involved.

Fire your judge – Most of us have tendency to scrutinize and negatively pre-judge any thoughts or ideas that are different. Much of this pre-judging comes from your associates but a major part of it comes from your own inner thinking. We are often our own worst critics! If you focus on all the reasons why a new idea *won't* work there is little possibility that it *will* work. So fire your judge, and the next time you come up with the seed of an idea ask yourself, "How can I make this work?"

Closely related to this thought is our fear of failure. It is often this fear that keeps us from thinking or trying new and different things. It is difficult for many of us to recognize the value of failure as Thomas Edison did when he said, "Every time I fail I've learned one more way not to achieve my goal." So, remember, most failures are just stepping stones to success.

Identify the rules and then break them – As a consultant on creative thinking in organizations I spent a lot of time helping my clients "break the rules". That was frightening to many because it is often imbued in us to "obey the rules". One of my favorite examples of this (I have lots of them) is the rule breaking that created the idea of hybrid vehicles. Years ago Audi questioned one of the basic rules of vehicle design – that a car has one engine. Breaking that relatively simple rule allowed them to think about the possibilities of having more than one engine, and the hybrid idea was born. Another example is *"the Fosbury flop."* For years high jumpers thought that they had to go over the high bar feet first. Then Dick Fosbury came along and changed everything by going over head first and the bar (so to speak) was reset.

So if you are thinking of expanding your thinking on a particular subject, start by identifying what specific rules shape your thinking, and then ask yourself what the possibilities would be if you were to break those rules.

Find your *Thinkorarium*

Glenn Curtiss, one of the most prolific inventors in the 1930's and 40s, had a cupola on top of his house overlooking one of the Finger Lakes in upstate New York. He called this his **thinkorarium** and it was where he went anytime he wanted to expand his thinking. Find a *thinkorarium* of your own (a garden spot, a comfortable chair in your music room, driving your car etc) where you can go and expand your thinking. Sometimes you just need a little of what I call, *soak time,* to help ideas develop fully. Let an idea mull over in your mind for a period of time and there's a good chance you'll discover some new connections that will help build on it.

Here are a few basic tips to bring out your creativity:

- Create a stretch vision of what you want.
- Try your best to be non-judgmental.

- Start from outrageous and work back. Practice *mental bungie jumping*.
- Examine and upset your thinking patterns often.
- Break the rules.
- Seek advice from others - especially those outside your expertise.
- Wonder a lot and let your ideas and thoughts marinate.
- If at first you don't succeed - give up - let go.
- Think in metaphors as much as you can.
- Laugh a lot and never lose touch with your sense of humor.

And always remember that **great ideas rarely enter the mind through the mouth**. Concentrate on listening intently to others, closely observing things around you, and building on the ideas that you take in.

Try some of these ideas now and let yourself go!

"You can never cross the ocean until you have the courage to lose sight of the shore."

Celery and Other Great Foods to Keep You Healthy

It's no secret that your diet is a critical part of staying young and healthy. Here are some foods that are super healthy for you that can help you lose weight and feel good. Celery comes out near the top of the list, but let's look at some others first.

Everyone knows that fruits are good for you, but certain fruits are super healthy and you should eat them often and substitute them for snacks wherever possible for a better diet. Oranges are really good for you. This is mainly due to the vitamin C content in them. They are also high in both antioxidants and fiber. All of this, and they taste great. Get in the habit of substituting oranges for some of those unhealthy snacks.

Bananas are also a brilliant food for your body. They are also very convenient, filling and portable. They are one of the best sources of potassium around and also contain plenty of fiber. If you tend to suffer from cramps now and then, which is quite common for seniors, they can help with this. If you don't feel like chomping on fruits you can always throw them into your Bullet and make a smoothie. I try to make fruit and veggie smoothies as a regular part of our diets (great lunches). Get yourself a **Bullet** to make it easy.

Nuts are really good for you despite their beautiful taste. Peanuts for example are high in nutrients as well as antioxidants and have been known to help people lose weight. However do not get this confused with peanut butter, which isn't too good for you.

Vegetables are another given; everybody knows that they are healthy. However one of the most overlooked but delicious and nutritious vegetable is broccoli. It contains both vitamins K and C, fiber, and a good amount of protein compared to other veggies.

If you are struggling for healthy options for your evening meal, have salmon. It is unbelievably tasty as well as being packed with nutrients. It contains vitamin D, Omega 3 and plenty of protein. Try it with some steamed veggies for a healthy but lovely dinner. Another option is tuna. Tuna can be eaten for lunch or dinner, contains plenty of protein, and next to no calories. And it is delicious in a salad.

Eggs are another option for you. They are packed with protein and also carry a very small calorific value. Eggs can be enjoyed as part of a salad or poached.

In terms of meats, your best bet is lamb, lean beef or chicken breast. Chicken breasts are very low in fat and calories but contain plenty of protein and other nutrients. So if in doubt, have some chicken.

Celery is probably something you either love or hate. I'm on the love side, and fondly remember our family snacking on celery sticks and Cheez Whiz (not sure about the Cheez Whiz). But here are some reasons that you should love it and make it a regular part of your meals and snacks. When you go to a party and there is an all you can eat buffet, you always see the untouched celery sitting next to the hummus and carrot sticks. I mean, who is going to chomp on celery when there are sandwiches and chicken wings up for grabs, right?

Well, next time you go to a party and see celery sticks, you should put a handful on your plate, and when you find out why – you will totally agree with me! Celery can in fact whiten your eyes, making them look brighter, tighter and much more youthful. As I'm getting a little older now, I'll try pretty much anything if it means I will look a little younger. Here's why this works.

Celery is jam packed full of vitamin A and just one large stalk of celery can deliver up to 10 percent of your daily need for Vitamin A. This is the group of nutrients that protects the eyes and prevents age-related degeneration of vision. Studies show that eating celery every day will in fact give you whiter, brighter eyes, and even accelerate your vision!

So why not give it a go? Celery also has lots more health benefits you probably aren't aware of too. For example, celery can help with bloating and it can reduce blood pressure, and detoxify your whole body. Not only that, but it is seriously low in calories with just 10 per stick! I don't know about you but the thought of just two stalks reducing your cholesterol by up to 7% is making me think I should be filling my frig with this stuff.

Celery is basically the food version of water, and everybody knows how good water is for you in every way imaginable. Helping your digestive system is just one of many advantages of including celery into your diet. Having high or heightened blood pressure can be very dangerous, so the fact that by just eating celery in your diet can help bring this down is something very useful to know.

20/20 Vision is something we could only dream about, until now! It's simple, just eat more celery and your eye health would never be at risk.

 Probably the main reason as to why people eat healthy foods is about weight loss. Celery is proven to keep you fuller for longer periods of time due to its water content. This results in your binging less on fattier foods.

Celery even makes you more mobile. Sports people and athletes eat plenty of celery to give them energy and help with water retention. It is so important to have regular PH levels in order to avoid acidic build up. A couple of sticks a day can ensure this alongside a nutritional balance diet.

Nobody enjoys being stressed. Is there anything that celery doesn't do? If you are having a bad day, just get a couple of celery sticks down you and it will all be fine. It will also help you sleep at night! Just when you thought you had heard it all. This green stick of pleasure will also improve your love life. **Get yourself to the grocery store immediately!**

We hear a lot in the press about what helps fight cancer and what you should stop doing in order to reduce the risk of cancer. But celery is one proven food which does delay the risk. So introduce it into your own diet and your family's diet as soon as possible. You can also blend it down into a juice.

So, if you like to snack and have a tendency to grab a bag of chips or cookies, go for some fruits or veggies instead. You may find them really enjoyable and they certainly will be much better for you.

"Don't let your mistakes wear you down. Place them under your feet and use them as stepping stones."

Proud Flesh

For those of you who have read some of my books, you know that I love stories that have deep meaning in our lives. I have shared many of them in past posts. American Indians tell wonderful stories and have some great words and phrases that often serve as powerful metaphors for many things. One such phrase is ***proud flesh***.

When a horse is injured, its flesh heals but there is always a reminder of the injury in the feelings (or perhaps lack of feelings) around the wound. Of course, this works for humans as well. Those who have ever had an operation, or received a deep cut know that the itching, strange pains, and numbness can last for a very long time – even after the wound is quite well healed.

I used this story in my book, **Surviving the Loss of Your Loved One: Jan's Rainbow**. This book was inspired by a rainbow that surrounded my home the day after I lost my wife of 40 years, Jan, to ovarian cancer. Losing a loved one can leave a very deep wound, and a very long-lasting scar. After the initial healing from the grieving process there will be some *proud flesh*. This *proud flesh* manifests itself as a setback in your own healing process. Just when you feel there is some light at the end of the tunnel of your healing, you regress into a few bad days. The wounds that you thought had healed begin to act up. My experience, and that of many of my associates in the bereavement process, is that this is quite common. And it often occurs after a year or so – just when you thought you were out of the woods. The good news is that the *proud flesh* usually doesn't act up for too long and that, after a while, the resulting pain is less severe.

I have lost a lot of other important people in my life and, with each loss there has been some *proud flesh*. And, of course, there are many other life events that can leave *proud flesh* as well. Think about the losses and other "wounds" you have received in your lifetime. Do you have any proud *flesh* as a result of these? I believe it is helpful to recognize this in our lives, and to work on dealing with the implications. Perhaps some of this *proud flesh* is still impacting your life. Recognizing its existence is the first step towards attaining long term healing.

Take some time and give this some serious thought. You may reveal a few things that are holding you back from living your life to the fullest. Good luck!

"As soon as you feel too old to do a thing – DO IT!"

Senior Swagger

I recently had the privilege of helping my friend, Joe Santoro, assemble his new book, **_Win The Biggest Game – Life._** This book focuses on helping younger people learn the skills necessary to become RICH and has 36 lessons to help them along this path. Joe's definition of RICH is:

"Someone who is healthy, knows who they are, is comfortable in their own skin, is doing what they like, is making enough money to support the lifestyle they desire, and has family and friends who love them and truly want to be with them".

One of the lessons deals with "Finding Your Swagger". When I think of swagger I think of Fonzie in "Happy Days". He walked with swagger, and he talked with swagger. I live in an area with a high density of seniors, and have spent some time observing them. I hate to admit it, but many seniors have lost their swagger. I'd love to see this change. Seniors actually have a lot to swagger about. Think of all the life skills they have amassed through the years.

In his book, Joe suggests that swagger is sort of a math equation:

High Self Esteem + High Self Confidence = Major Swagger

Self esteem is all about liking yourself. Do you like you? Start treating yourself like someone who is likeable, because deep down you are. Self confidence means believing in your skills. In your lifetime you have amassed a plethora of skills, many of which you probably don't even recognize. Take some time to enumerate these skills – it may surprise you how extensive they are.

Sometimes swagger is just believing you can learn to solve the problem, learn to hit the green, learn to make the moves, or even learn to say the right thing at the right time. So, what do you believe about YOU right now? That's the question. Do you believe in your skills? Do you believe you can learn new ones? Confidence is just believing, and here's why it's so important:

No one ever performs consistently at a level higher than what they believe to be true about themselves.

Come on, it's time to get a little more swagger.

"Whether you say, "I can" or you say, "I can't"...either way you're right"!

If I Had My Life to Live Over Again

If I had my life to live over again, I would _____. Have you ever asked yourself this question? They say "hindsight is 20/20" and, as I think more about it, there are so many things I would have done differently if I had known what I know now. Don't get me wrong – I've led what I would define as a pretty nice life, and I hope you feel the same about your own situation.

But as I think about it more deeply, I wonder how my life would be different if I had made some different decisions. I see a lot of folks in my age bracket that are much better off, much more fulfilled, and perhaps even much happier than I am. A lot of things have gone right for me – but not everything. Some were under my control, and some were not. I've lost a lot of loved ones in my life and sometimes I even wonder if I could have done something to change that. Most likely not, but that doesn't keep me from wondering.

My wife, Jan, was diagnosed with ovarian cancer in her forties. She was adamant about not wanting chemotherapy, and ended up relying on radiation treatments. She was declared cancer free, but several years later the cancer returned and I lost her. I have been dogged by the question ever since, "If I had insisted on her taking chemo treatments, would that have made a difference?"

But there are a lot less critical questions regarding things that I wish I had done:

- I wish I had taken my family on more trips.
- I wish I had experience more careers in my life.
- I wish I had taken up golf earlier in my life.
- I wish I had been developed stronger religious beliefs.
- What if I had made a career out of the US Army?
- And on and on.

What are some of the things on your list? For all those things that are on the list of things you wish you had done, there is one key question to ask:

WHAT IS KEEPING YOU FROM DOING THESE NOW?

Go through your list and work on how you can do some of the things now. It may not be too late!

"You are never too old to set another goal or dream a new dream."

A Few Ways You Can Supercharge Your Sense Of Humor

There are about 230 bones in your body, but the most important one of all is your "funny bone". In my book, _Add Humor To Your Life; Add Life To Your Humor,_ I share a lot of ways that you can use to raise your sense of humor. Here are a few of my favorites.

- **Start each day with a smile.** There are those of you who tend to wake up with a smile (me) and those who don't. The best way to start your day with a smile is to stand in front of your mirror and crack the biggest smile you can. Do this no matter how you feel. If you are feeling happy, you'll feel happier. If you feel lousy, I guarantee this will make you feel better. The person in the mirror will always be smiling back at you, so you're getting a double whammy here. I do this every morning and sometimes make a few silly faces at the dude in the mirror to boot.

- **Be someone's reason to smile each day.** Each day you should tell yourself that you are going to make someone smile. Often it doesn't take much – perhaps just a simple smile at someone you pass. A smile is such a powerful thing! It has a positive effect on both the giver and the receiver. The best candidates for a big smile are those you observe who just look unhappy (and my experience is that they are not too hard to find). A nice smile, along with a happy greeting may just turn their day around (and yours too).

- ☐ **Do something silly.** Every now and then we need to just really step outside of our normal behavior boxes, and do something silly. I'm reminded of one of my favorite books, _Totally Useless Skills,_ by Rick Davis. This is full of silly things to do. Or you may want to check out Monty Python's "Ministry of Silly Walks" on YouTube and try to invent some of your own walks. And there is also the book I wrote years ago, _Get Out Of Your Thinking Box_ which has 365 mostly silly things you can do to brighten your life and enhance your creativity.

- **Use "happy words".** The words we use are a reflection of how we feel and think. If we use "happy words", we will probably end up being "happy people". What kind of words do you tend to use? Take time sometime during your day to answer this question. Are the words you use in your normal conversation positive and happy? If not, takes steps change this. It will make a difference in helping you access your sense of humor.

- **Keep a "silly file".** For years I have kept track of all the things that tickled my funny bone. My file got so big that I actually turned it into a book, "**The Funniest Book You Will Ever Read**". The digital age made this so easy because so much of this material came to me via emails, social media etc. Whenever I came across something funny I would just "cut and paste" it to my "_Silly File_". Whenever I felt down I would go to this file, and it was just like getting a shot of "humor adrenalin". If you want a pre-made "_Silly File_" to start with, read my book (another shameless plug).

"Wrinkles should merely indicate where the smiles have been."

Mark Twain

The Four Seasons – A Wonderful Metaphor for Your Life

In the many years I spend in the northeast, I was always taken back by the beauty of autumn. One autumn, while on our annual leaf viewing trip, it occurred to me that the seasons provide us with a very interesting metaphor for life. Each season provides a different metaphorical twist to our thinking and, when we put these all together, the overall result is the opportunity to understand what you are going through in your life just a little bit better. Let's play with this one for a while.

Autumn is a time for shedding a lot of the well-rooted, mature ideas that have been adding color to our lives, but are getting tired. The great colors of summer give way to even more spectacular autumn colors. The falling leaves represent our ability to break current thinking patterns, and the ultimate composting of these leaves represents the great idea enhancing value that our combined experience and learning gives us.

The absence of leaves exposes the wonderful trunk and branch structure of the trees, which gives us a nice metaphor for the backbone of our thinking. If you were a child growing up in a seasonal climate you probably felt compelled to save a few of the more beautiful leaves and this is a good metaphor for building on some past idea nuggets.

The wonderful smell of autumn conjures up some of the most pleasant memories. For me these memories just seem to span my entire lifetime. I sometimes feel like a kid again, even though some people have told me that I've never stopped being a kid.

The **autumn season of the mind** is the time to challenge and shed old thinking and get reacquainted with the principles and values that support your thinking. It signals the time to question how events in your life impact the restructuring of your life in the future. What things need to really change in your life? What habits do you need to drop? What dreams do you have to reformulate? What current strengths do you need to nurture, and what new ones do you need to build for the future? What patterns of thinking do you need to change? Late autumn brings that first killing frost which ushers us into winter thinking.

Winter is a time for quiet thinking, contemplation, and introspection. As an author I find winter is my best time for writing and for generating some great new creative ideas. Deciduous trees, bulbs, and perennials are storing energy in their roots and gaining strength during the winter because they don't have to *show off* for a few months. A lot of our creative thinking is blocked by our need to *look good* and *show off*. Winter thinking suggests that we think below the surface without worrying about how we will be judged.

A blanket of snow just adds a little more security to protect those new, creative, and fragile ideas. As winter wears on, evergreens and the basic structure of trees that became exposed in the autumn can really strut their stuff. This is very well aligned with the idea that, after you set aside old patterns of thinking, some new, more creative thoughts are able to take shape. Since these are great metaphors for the basic principles and structures that guide our thinking, it helps us to stay in touch and build from them.

The winter season of the mind is the time for understanding the roots of your thinking and internally energizing the seeds of new ideas. Winter provides us with a few more questions to ask of ourselves. What do I have left to build on as I examine my basic structure? How might I turn my concerns and losses into something positive? This may seem like a strange question but, in my many years of studying creative thinking processes, I have found that there are always some positive aspects to even the most negative situations. What plans do you need to put in place for when the *spring* of your thinking arrives? What do you need to be doing to build up strength in your inner core?

And then comes **spring** when everything comes to life again. It's also a time for massive cleanup, as any gardener knows. It's also a very exciting time for gardeners because they are preparing for the beginning of a long period of growth as opposed to autumn when we prepare for a long period of rest. This is when new plants (ideas) really begin to grow and are nurtured along by warmer temperatures, longer days, and rain.

We rake, prune, cultivate, fertilize, plant, aerate, and mow because we know that whatever we do now will stick with us for a good part of the year. We also know that it will create healthier roots for new ideas in the future. What are some ways that you carry out these tasks to help new ideas grow?

The **spring season of the mind** is a time for growth and expansion of new ideas. It's a time for rekindling your excitement about living. The one thing that has always amazed me about spring is that it always seems to come. When I think of spring I think of the start of a new life. What new things do I need to plant in my life? What are some of the leftovers from winter that I need to clean up and throw out? What things do I need to *prune* in my new life? How might I cultivate and nurture new relationships that will make my new life more meaningful?

Summer is a time for harvesting and enjoying the fruits of our labor. For many it means vacation, a time to take your thinking to a more relaxing place and to view it from a different perspective. In winter thinking, the energy is concentrated below the surface at the root level. Summer thinking creates new ideas and expands on what is above the surface. We look at what we have and continually trim, prune, and deadhead to create more beauty.

The **summer season of the mind** is a time for improving and enjoying our ideas. Summer represents the beginning of feeling comfortable with your life. It may signal a time to move on and find new relationships and opportunities. How might I create lasting enjoyment in my next 50 years? What new opportunities can I grow in my life? How might I cultivate new relationships in my life?

Beethoven's Sixth Symphony (Pastoral) is all about the seasons. Listen to this while doing some deep thinking about the seasons of your life and it will greatly enhance the experience.

"Sometimes when you are in a dark place and you think you've been buried, you've really just been planted."

Managing Your Thoughts - The Story of Two Wolves

Our negative thoughts can create anxiety, anger, resentment, jealousy— an array of emotions. Negative thinking is normal. However, if this way of thinking becomes incessant, it can lead to depression and self-destructive behavior like addictions, derailing us from what we want most in life. At minimum, negative thinking saps our energy, erodes our self-confidence, and can put us in a bad mood. Certainly, many would agree that our thoughts co me and go so quickly that it's seems impossible to notice them. But with awareness and an attitude of self-compassion, we can redirect our negative thoughts to more positive ones.

Two Wolves is a Cherokee Indian legend and illustrates the most important battle of our lives – the one between our good and bad thoughts. Here is how the story goes:

An old Cherokee is teaching his grandson about life. "A fight is going on inside me," he said to the boy.

"It is a terrible fight and it is between two wolves. One is evil – he is anger, envy, sorrow, regret, greed, arrogance, self-pity, guilt, resentment, inferiority, lies, false pride, superiority, and ego." He continued, "The other is good – he is joy, peace, love, hope, serenity, humility, kindness, benevolence, empathy, generosity, truth, compassion, and faith. The same fight is going on inside you – and inside every other person, too."

The grandson thought about it for a minute and then asked his grandfather, "Which wolf will win?"

The old Cherokee simply replied, "The one you feed."

Our thoughts can be our own worst enemy. That is, if we let them. Think about how you may be "feeding" your negative thoughts by allowing them to rule your mind. Next time you have a negative thought, catch it and ask yourself, "What is this thought doing for me?" You will likely find that the answer is that all it is doing is disempowering you. You can immediately feel more empowered by focusing on something good in your life and cultivating the practice of gratitude.

We can create greater peace, confidence, and a more positive outlook by learning how to manage our thoughts. After all, this battle can be won because we have the power of choice!

"Which wolf are you feeding?" Remember, you always have a choice"!

"You are what you think."

Focusing On the Positive

In my observations of people through the years I have noticed that too many people tend to focus on all the reasons why things *can't be* done. As someone once said, *"Where there's a will there's a won't."* And then there are those of us who focus on how things *can be* done. I've always tried my best to be one of them – and you should too. I realize of course that there is a continuum here, and most people's thinking doesn't occur on either end, but somewhere between the two extremes. I've come to believe that the norm tends to be further towards the "can't be" end and, when the focus is on the reasons why things can't be done, it is likely nothing will get done.

I'm reminded of a story I heard quite a while ago that has rather stuck with me through the years:

It was Christmas and a little boy and girl were very excited to see what Santa had left so they snuck down a little early to take a peak. The only thing they saw was a huge pile of manure next to the tree. The little boy ran back to his room crying thinking that he must have behaved very badly to deserve this. The little girl ran to the woodshed to get a shovel, came back and began shoveling like mad saying. "There must be a pony in here somewhere."

Now this may not be the most exciting analogy, but sometimes I think you need to shovel a little manure out of the way if you want to find the things you want in your life.

If you can focus on how things "can be done" there is a much higher probability that you will get results. In my creative problem solving consulting I often used a technique from my friend, Sidney Shore, called, "What's good about it?" When you encounter a problem, focus on the things that are good about that problem, and use these things to help solve the problem. It may surprise you to learn that there are always more positive aspects of a negative situation than you thought there were. And this will push you into focusing on the positive.

If you think you may be one of those who lean toward a negative focus you may have to work on moving to the positive side. Try it out on the next few problems or decision points you encounter. This may be a bit uncomfortable at first, but push as hard as you can into a positive focus. Enlist the help of someone close to you if necessary. Once you are able to regularly focus on the positive you'll be a much happier, more productive person. And, if you have some friends or associates that tend toward the negative, try to push them to the positive. In doing this you will also strengthen your own ability to stay positive.

It's important to note that the words you use have an impact upon your ability to focus on the positive. If you use positive words you will find it much easier to have a positive outlook. If you use negative words you may find it difficult to stray from negative thought. Think about the words you tend to use. Track them for a while if you can. Do you lean towards positive or negative words? If you lean towards the negative, make a concerted effort to add more positive words to your vocabulary. It will definitely change your outlook!

Some of my friends consider me to be the ultimate optimist. One of my inspirations comes from an article I found in the newspaper years ago about Les Paul, the guitar genius. Here are some highlights from that article that should also inspire you to focus on the positive:

When Paul performs on the electric guitar it's hard to believe that acute arthritis has immobilized all the fingers of his right hand and crippled all but two fingers on his left, or fingerboard, hand. "I had to learn to play the guitar all over again as the arthritis got worse," Paul says. "I play real good now with just two fingers."

Paul also suffers from the effects of a 1948 automobile accident where he suffered a broken back, fractured pelvis, broken collarbone, broken ribs, a ruptured spleen, and a right arm that was so crushed there was talk of amputating it. Doctors managed to reconstruct his arm and set it pointed at his navel, in a guitar-playing position. "It won't move but I can still hold a guitar," Paul says with a laugh.

He has also been through bone-graft surgery on his left hand; he has suffered from sciatica and Meniere's disease; he has had three operations on his right ear to correct a broken eardrum; and has had a quintuple heart bypass. Nevertheless, Paul has managed to put a positive spin on his misfortunes.

"With every setback, every hospitalization, I've done some creating," he says. "If you can't play, you can think, you can sit there and invent. So when someone tells me I've had a lot of hardships I tell them that a lot of good things have come from them."

If that story doesn't inspire you to be an optimist, nothing will! By the way, I've noticed that *Optimist's Clubs* are popping up in a number of places (such as where I live in The Villages, Florida). If there is one near you consider joining it.

"Happy people focus on what they have.

Unhappy people focus on what's missing,"

The Mind and Body Challenge

The way I look at it, our bodies, and our brains are designed as working machines. If you don't keep them working, and continually challenge them, they will just atrophy and rust. "Challenge" is the keyword here, and I believe you need to exercise both your body and brain to just past the "comfort zone" to get maximum benefit. Any exercise is good, but the best exercise is to work to the end of your comfort zone – and then add a little more. Like a good sports car, you need to take it into the "red zone' every now and then. You need to know when to stop though, because you shouldn't overdo it.

It's all a matter of getting into a few habits. For your physical health, get into the habit of walking, swimming, golfing, racket sports (tennis, pickle ball, racquetball etc.), biking, or just working out. Stick to it and have fun with it. Remember, those *abs of steel* are probably not coming back, and you're not exactly trying out for the Olympics. Your goal is to just keep your mind and body healthy.

To keep yourself mentally challenged, get into the habit of engaging in something that stretches your thinking every day. First thing in the morning is always a good time for this. I think of these challenges as being in four categories:

Word Challenges

This includes crosswords, *Words With Friends*, and *Word Search*, along with others. There are scads of crossword books and apps available, or you might just get in the habit of solving those in your local newspaper. Most of the time, they start with a fairly easy one on Monday, and get progressively more difficult each day. *Words with Friends* is a rather addictive game of Scrabble that you play on line with friends. It's a fun, challenging way to sharpen you connection with words. Download it and challenge a few of your friends, I guarantee you'll love it.

Visual Challenges

Jigsaw Puzzles and those that ask you to spot the difference between 2 pictures are my favorites. My favorite jigsaw app is called *Magic World*, which you can download for free.

Logic

Sudoku is the overall favorite here. There are dozens of books and some very good apps that can provide you with challenges at every level. If you are new to this, start at an easy level and work yourself up to one that really challenges you. My favorite *Sudoku* app is called *Finger Arts* which you can also download for free.

Memory

And then there pure memory games like *Trivial Pursuit* and *Are You Smarter Than a Fifth Grader?* There are a number of apps for both of these if you search for them. Or you may want to challenge your friends or family in a board game that focuses on memory.

And, if you want some more mental challenges, buy one of the numerous brain games books which are full of some very different challenges at all levels.

OK – get up and have at it!

"The older you get, the more important it is not to act your age."

Health Benefits of Being Nice – Random Acts of Kindness

Small acts of kindness and generosity can actually make you a healthier person and change your life. Being kind to others can actually pay you back in the form of major health benefits. It also leaves a positive mark on the lives of others and can make you feel great. Being kind to others rewards the human brain with a release of feel-good hormones that can result in a lowering of blood pressure, reduced heart rate, and a feeling of contentment.

You don't have to give someone the coat off your back to show you care. Regardless of where you live, how much you earn, or how much time you have, there are infinite ways to choose kindness. And they all count.

Here are a few random acts of kindness to make somebody's day:

1. **Smile at everyone you see (especially strangers).**

   Smiling is contagious. Research shows that to better understand one another, humans are programmed to mimic the expressions of others. So when you smile at someone, they'll have a hard time not smiling back. Even if they're faking it, they'll still benefit. The best folks to smile at might be those who look stressed or cranky (sometimes not hard to find).

2. **Pick up the tab for the person behind you**

   This one works great at the coffee shop (not so much at a BMW dealership). For just a few bucks, you'll make someone's day, and inspire others in line to pay it forward too. That's because witnessing a kind act elicits an emotion called "elevation," which increases motivation to help others.

3. **Help out around your neighborhood**

   Have you ever noticed that those neighbors who help others seem to be happy themselves? Older adults who donated more time are happier and healthier than those who give less or none at all. Small acts of help are fine (you don't have to paint their house). Simply being of service is enough to garner health benefits.

   People who have a sense of belonging and feel connected to their communities are more likely to report better physical health than those with less "social capital," a term sometimes used to describe feelings of trust, cooperation, and working toward a greater good. So, the next time you see a neighbor working on something, ask if you can help.

4. **Give a compliment**

How often do you praise someone in your head, but never actually tell them how much you admire their fashion sense, their gardens, or their cooking? Speak up! It's like handing over a wad of cash, according to a Japanese study. When researchers doled out compliments as rewards for a job well done, they found that it activated the striatum, the region of the brain that lights up when you find money.

5. **Pay attention to your partner**

Americans check their smart phones morning, noon, and night — an average of 47 times per day. Your goal for tonight: 0.

All the time we spend with technology is hurting our relationships. In a 2016 survey of 143 married or cohabiting women, the majority admitted that their devices regularly interrupt quality leisure time, mealtimes, conversations, and other interactions with their partners.

This has been linked to relationship discontent, depression, and general dissatisfaction with life. Not only will you and your partner feel more connected after a night without screens, but research suggests you'll sleep better, too.

6. **Do something really special for your family**

Most of us get stuck in our routines and don't often go out of our way to try something different. So why not surprise your family with something different? Cook them a very special meal, take them to a nice restaurant, buy them all gifts, take them on a trip, or just go for a nice drive. Doing nice things for loved ones makes you feel warm and fuzzy

7. **Ask an friend or associate about his or her weekend**

If you spend time in an office environment, whether it's full-time or as a volunteer, take time to chat up with a newbie — or someone who doesn't have a ton of office pals. Having a friendly, supportive workplace can help you and your associates live longer. If you have a friend or neighbor who doesn't have someone to chat with on a regular basis, go out of your way to chat with them. You'll make them (and yourself) feel good and perhaps learn a lot too.

In other words, a simple 'Hi' could save a life. You often think it. Now say it and change the world.

"Those who bring sunshine into the lives of others
cannot keep it from themselves."

A Very Funny Look at Aging

I have been teaching a few courses at The Villages Enrichment Academy based on three of my books. These courses are designed to provide seniors with some sage advice on how to stay young. If time permits, I usually share a very entertaining video that takes a humorous look at aging. The most entertaining video I have is from Fritz Coleman, a weather-caster for NBC in San Diego, and his presentation at the Pasadena Conference on Aging. He probably has a little time on his hands since the weather forecast there is about the same every day.

This guy is just incredibly funny, and people love the video. His views on aging are just a gas and I know it will make your day! Share it with your friends; they will love you for it. Just Google "Fritz Coleman on Aging" and check it out.

By the way, I find that leading these courses has been a wonderful way for me to stay on track with my own learning. Also, I will venture a guess that just about all of you who are reading this have the knowledge and capacity to teach some courses of your own. Is there an adult learning center somewhere near you? Do you have some topic(s) that may qualify you as somewhat of an expert? (of course you do).

If you are not sure, you may want to start by taking some of the courses offered by a continuing education organization near you. It's never too late to pour some more stuff into that brain of yours. Your brain will love you for it! After taking a few of these courses you may get the bug to take on one of your own.

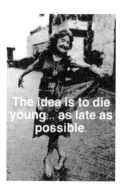

"There are seven days in a week and "someday" isn't one of them".

Helping Others / Helping Yourself

This is one of my favorite stories about the value of helping others. There's a great lesson in this story – what goes around, comes around. Always keep an eye out for someone you can help. Helping others is one of the best ways I know to feel good about yourself.

One day a man saw an old lady, stranded on the side of the road, but even in the dim light of day, he could see she needed help. So he pulled up in front of her Mercedes and got out. His Pontiac was still sputtering when he approached her.

Even with the smile on his face, she was worried. No one had stopped to help for the last hour or so. Was he going to hurt her? He didn't look safe; he looked poor and hungry. He could see that she was frightened, standing out there in the cold. He knew how she felt. It was those chills which only fear can put in you. He said, "I'm here to help you, ma'am. Why don't you wait in the car where it's warm? By the way, my name is Bryan Anderson."

Well, all she had was a flat tire, but for an old lady, that was bad enough. Bryan crawled under the car looking for a place to put the jack, skinning his knuckles a time or two. Soon he was able to change the tire. But he had to get dirty and his hands hurt.

As he was tightening up the lug nuts, she rolled down the window and began to talk to him. She told him that she was from St. Louis and was only just passing through. She couldn't thank him enough for coming to her aid.

Bryan just smiled as he closed her trunk. The lady asked how much she owed him. Any amount would have been all right with her. She already imagined all the awful things that could have happened had he not stopped. Bryan never thought twice about being paid. This was not a job to him. This was helping someone in need, and God knows there were plenty, who had given him a hand in the past. He had lived his whole life that way, and it never occurred to him to act any other way.

He told her that if she really wanted to pay him back, the next time she saw someone who needed help, she could give that person the assistance they needed, and Bryan added, "And think of me." He waited until she started her car and drove off. It had been a cold and depressing day, but he felt good as he headed for home, disappearing into the twilight.

A few miles down the road the lady saw a small cafe. She went in to grab a bite to eat, and take the chill off before she made the last leg of her trip home. It was a dingy looking restaurant. Outside were two old gas pumps. The whole scene was unfamiliar to her. The waitress came over and brought a clean towel to wipe her wet hair. She had a sweet smile, one that even being on her feet for the whole day couldn't erase.

~ 32 ~

The lady noticed the waitress was nearly eight months pregnant, but she never let the strain and aches change her attitude. The old lady wondered how someone who had so little could be so giving to a stranger. Then she remembered Bryan.

After the lady finished her meal, she paid with a hundred dollar bill. The waitress quickly went to get change for her hundred dollar bill, but the old lady had slipped right out the door. She was gone by the time the waitress came back. The waitress wondered where the lady could be. Then she noticed something written on the napkin.

There were tears in her eyes when she read what the lady wrote: "You don't owe me anything. I have been there too. Somebody once helped me out, the way I'm helping you. If you really want to pay me back, here is what you do, do not let this chain of love end with you." Under the napkin were four more $100 bills.

Well, there were tables to clear, sugar bowls to fill, and people to serve, but the waitress made it through another day. That night when she got home from work and climbed into bed, she was thinking about the money and what the lady had written. How could the lady have known how much she and her husband needed it? With the baby due next month, it was going to be hard... She knew how worried her husband was, and as he lay sleeping next to her, she gave him a soft kiss and whispered soft and low, "Everything's going to be all right. I love you, Bryan Anderson."

That's nice, isn't it? Keep this story in mind the next time you get a chance to help someone.

"Life is not measured by the number of breathes we take, but by the moments that take our breath away."

The Nature and Forms of Humor

Humor is very contagious, and it's something that you want to catch. It spreads quite easily, and is pretty much the same across all cultures. There are very few situations where humor is not appropriate and valuable. Some would say that funerals are one of those situations, but I have been a part of many of these, and I can say that humor almost always played a part in making them easier. One of the most interesting characteristics of humor involves a *chicken vs. the egg question*. **Am I happy because I'm laughing, or am I laughing because I'm happy?**

We know that laughing and smiling has wonderful beneficial effects, but your body doesn't know whether you are laughing at something that struck you funny, or just laughing for no reason at all. This has some interesting implications on how you can use humor in your life. You don't always have to wait for something to make you laugh or smile - just do it and you'll feel better! Start each day by smiling at yourself in the mirror. I guarantee the person in the mirror will smile back at you. Laugh at that person in the mirror and he/she will laugh along with you.

They say that babies laugh over 300 times per day, and the normal adult only a handful of times. So we were all born with the ability to laugh at about everything. This ability sometimes erodes through the years. Here is a YouTube that has had something like 100 million hits, and I think you will see why. Watch this whenever you need a little humor boost. Just Google:

Baby Laughing at Ripping Paper

Humor can come in several forms and here are just a few:

- Jokes
- Quotes and Quips
- Pleasant incongruities
- Cartoons
- Spaced Out Stuff - Exaggerations

Jokes are probably one of the most popular and most used forms - but perhaps not always the best. One reason is that they often take victims. If you use an ethnic group, or lawyers, or blondes as the butt of your joke, not everyone will find it funny. And you could really alienate some folks. Since some of these jokes are quite funny, and I choose to use humor only in positive ways, I get around this problem using myself as the butt of the joke (How many *old guys* does it take to_____?).

I could go on and on explaining the different forms, but I have promised to keep these posts short. In my book, **Add Humor To Your Life; Add Life To Your Humor,** I explain these forms in detail with many examples (a shameless plug).

"The world always looks brighter from behind a smile."

~ 34 ~

What's Love Got To Do With It?

Does love really make the world go around? Maybe not, but it sure makes the world a better place to live. While on a speaking engagement in South Africa I became aware of one of the most interesting concepts ever. That concept is **Ubuntu.** The dictionary defines this as the quality made up of sympathy, kindness, and respect toward other people that is considered to be a part of the African way of life.

In Archbishop Desmond Tutu's words:

"A person with Ubuntu is open and available to others, affirming of others, does not feel threatened that others are able and good, based from a proper self-assurance that comes from knowing that he or she belongs in a greater whole and is diminished when others are humiliated or diminished, when others are tortured or oppressed".

Don't be afraid to tell your spouse, children, grandchildren, family and friends that you love them. And don't be afraid to fall in love with them a little more each day. Laugh with them as much as you can. As Victor Borge says, *"Laughter is the shortest distance between two people."* And don't be afraid to cry with them as well in circumstances that call for it. If you have pets show them as much love as you can – they always eat that up. And a wagging tail or soft purr is a great stress reducer. Maybe God should have given us the power to purr or tails to wag.

And don't be afraid to show some affection to those you interact with each day even if it is just giving them a nice smile and wishing them a good day. Smiling at total strangers can make you both feel good. And don't worry about the one out of every hundred who may consider you a pervert.

Hugging is a great way to solidify relationships. Never pass up an opportunity to hug family and friends. You might be surprised how much most people enjoy a good hug. I think that among those who love to be hugged are nurses. I have an incredible respect for nurses and will always hug any nurse that assists me to show my appreciation.

And never pass up an opportunity to shake the hand of a service man or women in the airport or any place else that you happen to spot them. Thank them for their service. It'll make them feel good – and it will make you feel good too. We can never show enough appreciation to those who serve their country. And while you are at it you might want to consider thanking a police officer, fire fighter, EMT or teacher. Some of these people put their lives on the line every day for you.

Extend a hand and help others out whenever you can, even if they are total strangers. If you are able, look into ways you can volunteer your time to helping others. While you're at it, call up some of your old friends and tell them you've been thinking about them.

Times flies, and it is very easy to lose touch with old friends. Don't let that happen. Try to get in touch with an old friend at least once a week. Also, go out of your way to maximize your relationships with family members, no matter how far away they are.

Surround yourself with things you love (music, plants, pictures, keepsakes, hobbies etc.). This will help you to continually stay connected to those things that are important in your life.

Life is too short to waste on hating anyone or anything. I believe that most of us have built up fairly long lists of things or people that we dislike. As a matter of fact, many of our world problems exist because of long-standing biases and hatred that some have towards other people. Try to make friends with someone who you have not cared for in the past. It may not always work but, if it helps you create a new friend, it will make you feel good. There is a double benefit here – you get the plus from creating a new friend and you eliminate a minus that you may have been carrying around for a while.

"Being deeply loved by someone gives you strength,
while loving someone deeply gives you courage."
Lao Tzu

"Where there is love there is life."
Mahatma Gandhi

The Mayonaise Jar

As I've mentioned before. I have long been a collector of stories that have great life messages. The story of the *Mayonnaise Jar* is one of them. Read it carefully at least twice, and think about what this might mean in your own situation. I think you'll find it will stimulate a lot of very powerful thoughts. It always does for me.

Once in a while, you'll come across a story that makes you think. The simple story of the professor with the mayonnaise jar and two cups of coffee is one of those gems. The origin of the story is unknown, and different variations of it exist online. We may never find out who wrote this inspiring tale or if it even happened in real life, but we can definitely learn some valuable lessons from reading it. Here is the story in its entirety:

When things in your lives seem almost too much to handle, when 24 hours in a day are not enough, remember the mayonnaise jar and the two cups of coffee.

A professor stood before his philosophy class and had some items in front of him. When the class began, he wordlessly picked up a very large and empty mayonnaise jar and proceeded to fill it with golf balls. He then asked the students if the jar was full. They agreed that it was.

The professor then picked up a box of pebbles and poured them into the jar. He shook the jar lightly. The pebbles rolled into the open areas between the golf balls. He then asked the students again if the jar was full. They agreed it was.

The professor next picked up a box of sand and poured it into the jar. Of course, the sand filled up everything else. He asked once more if the jar was full. The students responded with an unanimous "yes."

The professor then produced two cups of coffee from under the table and poured the entire contents into the jar, effectively filling the empty space between the sand. The students laughed.

"Now," said the professor as the laughter subsided, "I want you to recognize that this jar represents your life. The golf balls are the important things — your family, your children, your health, your friends and your favorite passions — and if everything else was lost and only they remained, your life would still be full. The pebbles are the other things that matter like your job, your house and your car. The sand is everything else — the small stuff.

"If you put the sand into the jar first," he continued, "there is no room for the pebbles or the golf balls. The same goes for life. If you spend all your time and energy on the small stuff you will never have room for the things that are important to you.

"Pay attention to the things that are critical to your happiness. Play with your children. Take time to get medical checkups. Take your spouse out to dinner. Play another 18. There will always be time to clean the house and fix the disposal. Take care of the golf balls first — the things that really matter. Set your priorities. The rest is just sand."

One of the students raised her hand and inquired what the coffee represented.

The professor smiled. "I'm glad you asked. It just goes to show you that no matter how full your life may seem, there's always room for a couple of cups of coffee with a friend."

What are the "*golf balls*" of your life? Are you taking care of these? What can you do re-arrange some of your priorities so that *golf balls, pebbles, and sand* of your life are taken care of in the appropriate order? And, are you leaving enough space in your schedule to have a couple of cups of coffee with some friends from time to time?

"In the end it's not the years in your life that count. It's the life in your years."

Abraham Lincoln

Fitness Trackers

Perhaps one of the hottest selling family of products today is that of fitness trackers. My first one was a **FitBit Charge** which, unfortunately, is now somewhere on a beach on Grand Bahama Island. I now have a **Garmin Vivosmart HR** which I really love. Both of these products are very nice, but there is a plethora of these fitness trackers available. Visit your local Best Buy and you'll see an entire aisle dedicated to them. Better still visit Amazon.com , search "fitness trackers" and see what pops up. You'll be amazed, and you'll probably be confused as well. But I think everyone, especially those in the over 55 crowd, should have one of these. And, by the way, it's a great idea for a gift for those you care about.

There are easily a dozen or more different brands, and prices ranging from $10 to $150 or so. One of the things offered with the better known brands is the ability to sync to your other devices (smart phones, PC's, laptops, IPods etc.). I think this is an important thing to consider since it allows you to track some good health data over time. By the way, it also tracks your sleeping habits, how long you sleep, and how well you sleep.

I would probably stay away from the real cheap brands which might be disappointing. Sticking with Garmin or FitBit is probably a good choice. These both include rather attractive supporting apps to let you track results over time. I'm not sure about the other brands.

So what do these little marvels do? My Garmin tracks and displays my steps, calories, distance, floors climbed, intensity minutes, calories burned, and heart rate. What makes it even handier is that it defaults back to time and date – so you can give your watch a rest. I would recommend having a tracker with a heart rate monitor. It never hurts to see what your pulse is, especially during exercise. When synced to my smart phone, it also displays calls, texts, social, music, games etc. with vibration beats.

So put this on your wish list or just go out and get one for yourself. And, while you are at it, get one for your significant other too. You can thoroughly entertain each other every night by comparing steps, calories burned, hours of sleep etc. The older we get, the easier we are to entertain.

"To be old and wise you first have to be young and stupid."

Writing Your Life Story

Writing a life story can be a great experience. I worked almost a year on mine and enjoyed every minute of it. Initially I did it because I thought my children, and grandchildren, would like to know what it was like in the generation before them. I sure would have loved it if I could have read some life stories from my parents and grandparents. When you leave this earth all of your history goes with you unless you take the time to leave some here. I think that is one of the key reasons why I am so addicted to writing. I've lived a pretty interesting life and been able to amass a pretty good base of knowledge in a number of areas. Why should I take this with me without sharing it first with as many people as I can?

I started writing my life story by going back as far as I could remember and sort of rambling forward from there. But I found that the more I brought out from my active memory bank, the more I was able to dig deeper into my memory and remember things that I had long ago forgotten. This was a great learning experience for me. Reliving most of my experiences was fun. Reliving some of the more tragic experiences sometimes brought tears to my eyes but, in the end, made me feel like I had unloaded some baggage, and that's always a good thing. Based on my experience here are a few tips on how to create your life story.

Start by separating your life into different eras that represent the parts of your life that were most important. I separated mine into:

- The early years
- High school years
- College years
- Marriage and Beginning a Family
- My Army Years
- My Career with Kodak
- Building a Home and Growing a Family
- Early Retirement and a New Career
- Loss of my wife – Jan
- My Second Chance at Love – Jean
- Where I am Now

For each of these eras I began by brainstorming the events that came to mind. I then repeated this process several times until I couldn't think of anything else to enter. That gave me a good starting point to begin embellishing my thoughts for each of the categories. This was a wonderful experience because, the more I wrote, the more great thoughts from the past came to mind.

And then to spice things up a bit I added newsflashes from certain key turning points in my life (when I was born, graduations, military service, building a home etc.). Doing this was a blast! For example here is the newsflash for the year I was born. You can easily find this information at various websites such as **peoplehistory.com**

Newsflash! It's 1941. Franklin Delanor Roosevelt is president. The war in Europe is dominating world affairs. On December 7th the US is attacked by the Japanese in Pearl Harbor and we enter into WW2. The average cost of a house is $4,075, average wages are $1750 per year, a gallon of gas is 12 cents, average price of a new car is $850, and average house rent is $32 per month. Mount Rushmore is completed and a bill is passed to make the 4th Thursday in November Thanksgiving Day. On my birthday the Boston Bruins sweep the Detroit Redwngs to win the Stanley Cup.

I also included lots of pictures in the story. I spent hours digitizing pictures from my childhood days going back to my great grandparents in the 1800's who I never even knew (I'm not that old!). The pictures really make the story interesting, and the process of going through and scanning them was an experience in itself. During this process I was able to gain a lot of information for building my family tree. Working on your family tree is something you may want to consider along with writing your life story. There is some nice family tree software available and ancestry.com is a wonderful source of information.

I concluded by sharing my philosophy on life and a summary of some of the things that are important to me including:

- The high points of my life
- The low points of my life
- My favorite songs
- All of the cars I have owned
- All of the Presidents during my years (along with a brief impression of each one)
- Our family pets
- My religious and political beliefs

I didn't have the luxury of having family members that I could talk with who could add some ideas since my whole family has passed. But I would suggest that you interact with as many members of your family as you can to get their input. If you have some family members that are along in years do it while you have the chance. My experience is that for the most part, they love to share this information.

You may also want to have yearly updates and leave an open chapter or two. I'm thinking of a chapter called *my hundredth birthday,* and perhaps one about *my second millennium.* Yes – it's good to be an optimist! Have fun!

"A diamond is a chunk of coal that did well under pressure."

Be a 'Glutton for Funishment'

What on earth is a "glutton for funishment"? It is someone who just sees the humor in everything around him or her. When you take everything around you lightly, it's easy to find something humorous about nearly everything you see or hear. And, if something doesn't pop up right away, then look a little deeper. As I am writing this I am looking out the window of our Upstate New York summer place which is in a very nice spot on the edge of the woods. I'm watching 2 chipmunks chase each other around the yard and I am being thoroughly entertained. My day may be brighter because of these two *cuties*.

And as I am watching this my thoughts go to many years ago when my sister and brother and I would chase each other around our yard. Many of the ideas and techniques in my book, ***Add Humor To Your Life; Add Life To Your Humor***, are designed to make you a better "glutton for funishment". But it starts with your ability to see humor in just about everything.

Here are a couple of examples I recall from my own experience. One day I was driving to a meeting at a satellite plant along a highway that had just been striped. I was looking at the new yellow stripe along the shoulder, and there was a dead raccoon right on the line that had just been painted over with the stripe. Maybe that's not that funny (certainly not for the raccoon) but I couldn't stop laughing to myself. I think I even used this story to illustrate a point during our meeting.

While waiting in my doctor's office for an appointment one day, I was checking out the various leaflets on display. One of them was titled, "You and Dandruff" and it really got me going. It just struck me so funny that a brochure on dandruff would be in a doctor's office which I'm sure had some more important things to deal with. You see, you CAN find humor in almost any situation.

So, today, take a different look at everything you see, and try to find something funny about it. It helps to be smiling while you do this, just to put you in the right frame of mind. You may be surprised at what you find. Then try to make a habit of doing this whenever you can. Enjoy the experience!

"It's never too late to have a happy childhood. You are only young once, but you can be immature all your life

Walking

It's pretty obvious that physical and mental activities are great contributors to long, happy lives. Walking is one of the easiest and best things you can do to stay physically active. Committing to a walking regimen is pretty easy to do.

They say 10,000 steps per day is a good goal to aim for. Sounds like a lot, doesn't it? If you are not used to walking, I wouldn't suggest starting with this many steps. Start with a mile walk, and work your way up from there. A 10,000 step walk is about 5 miles. There are some nice gadgets that will help you with this program. If you have a smart phone, IPad, or similar device, go to the app store and search for pedometers and see what you find. Most of these are free, and work quite well. A good selection of pedometers can also be found at sports stores like Dick's.

And a fitness band is always a good choice for tracking your progress. Get one that can be paired to your smart phone so you can track your progress over time. You may also want one that will give you heart rate and blood pressure readings so you can see what's going on during your walk.

Here are a few tips to help you with your walking regimen:

- Mix up your walking locations so you don't get bored. Walking around the neighborhood can get old after a while. We spend our summers at an RV Resort on New York's Erie Canal. You could walk from Albany to Buffalo if you wanted to. But we sometimes take short drives to different starting points just to mix it up. Are there some parks near you? Try walking them. Weather bad? The malls are great walking areas.
- If you are a golfer, walk the course every now and then.
- If there are some places you go that are within walking range, walk instead of drive.
- Walk a treadmill when possible. This can get rather boring, but you can catch up on your reading at the same time.
- Get into the habit of walking the same time each day. I find that early morning is most often the best time, especially during the summer heat.
- Try the get your significant other to walk with you. It gives you someone to talk with and, of course, helps them out too.

Whenever I visit my cardiologist, the first question he asks me is, "Have you been walking"? Walking is great for the heart. I must admit that after each walk I just feel much better. So — get out there and start walking!

"Every great oak was once a nut that stood its ground."

Grandfather Was a Very Wise Man

I am probably repeating myself, but I love stories that contain deep meanings for life. I used this story often in my presentations on creative thinking. It's such a powerful message! Read it over a few times and let it sink in. How might this thought impact your life? I think you may find some interesting answers that could provide new opportunities to influence your future. Share this post with your friends if you can too.

You have the opportunity to make transformational changes in your life and in the lives of others. But sometimes these changes are not made in leaps and bounds but are the additive result of the small steps you take. The following story appeared several years ago in our local paper and was written by an American Indian by the name of R.C. Dana. It has been on my mind and guided me through much of my thinking in these past few years. I hope you find just as powerful.

Many years ago, a young man and his grandfather spent their days together, as was the custom. The old man spent much time teaching the boy how to hunt, fish, and make things, and to do it all in a sacred way. Having lived many years, the grandfather possessed many great powers of healing and teaching. Great was his knowledge of many things. One day the grandfather said to the boy, "We will change the course of the mighty river."

The boy was filled with wonder, for he knew that his grandfather was a great man and could do great things. But change the course of a great river? Who of mortal man could accomplish such a great deed?

As they approached the river, the boy's heart leapt as he imagined the course of the river being changed. When they got to the bank of the river, the old man reached down into the river and picked out a rock about the size of a melon. The boy watched as the hole that the rock left began to fill with water, and he understood that in some small way the old man had indeed changed the course of the mighty river.

The old man looked at the boy with a twinkle in his eye and said, "This is the way the great river is changed, one rock at a time. It is the duty of every man who walks to change the course of rivers. Every action that you do, every word that you say will affect or change the course of a person's life. Keep on changing the course of rivers, little one." Grandfather was a wise man.

"You can't start the next chapter of your life if you keep re-reading the last one."

What Makes You Essential?

One of the key things that will help you to lead a happy life is knowing that you have a strong reason for being – a feeling that you are essential. So what does make you essential? Who are the people that rely on you? What are the skills that you have and can build on? What are your goals in life? What are the things in your life you have left to do? When I lost my wife, Jan, I decided that my extensive knowledge in creative thinking could be put to use to help others cope with loss in their life. And now I'm using these same ideas to help people grow older in style.

You don't think anything makes you essential? Think again. Write down all the possibilities and expand on them. These don't have to be things that change the world, just things that help you realize that you are important, and maybe play a major role in the lives of your friends, family, and others. And remember, as someone once said,

> *"If you think you're too small to make a difference then you've never been in bed with a mosquito."*

To really expand your thinking in this area, start your own company, and hire yourself on as President and CEO. Here's your chance to have that great title! You may even want to create a business card to hand out to your friends and family. Your company could be **Me Inc,** and you can give yourself any title you want. Better still; give your company a really creative name! Here are a few possibilities for your title

Raging Inexorable Thunder-Lizard Creativity Evangelist

All That Is Powerful and Wise

Big Kahuna

Director of Fun

Master of Madness

Pride Piper of Creativity

Wicked Good Idea Generator

Idea Gooser

Wizard of Wonder

Hope Builder

Cerebral Proctologist

Chief Imagination Officer

Human Being

Director of Everything

Chief Humor Officer

Squeezer of Organizational Thinking Juices

Manager of Mischief

Rocker of Boats

Feel free to use any of these or, better still, invent your own title, one that really turns you on and excites you. Use any of these titles as stepping stones to create your own. And you don't have to keep the same title forever. Change to a new title whenever you want – remember you are your own boss. Finding out what makes you essential creates a powerful incentive to lead you on the way to a long, happy life.

"The road to success is always under construction."

"Be what you is, not what you ain't. Cause if you is what you ain't, you ain't what you is."

This is one of my favorite all-time quotations from an old time jazz musician (whose name I have forgotten). Read it over a few times and its meaning will grow on you.

Is Drinking Water the Secret to Long Life?

I have long known that drinking water is important to keeping your weight down, but there are so many other benefits. It seems like a real no-brainer – drinking water is just not that difficult. They say eight 8-ounce glasses a day is about the right amount. Should you choose tap water, purified water, or ionized water? If the quality of your tap water is good then that may be the best choice, and cheapest way to go too.

Some people seem to be obsessed with bottled water. But I think this is an expensive option (to say nothing about the terrible impact of our environment). And I have friends who claim ionized water has changed their lives. My preference is filtered water from my fridge. The important thing is to get in the habit of drinking the minimum amount per day.

How does water affect your health?

Here are just a few positive outcomes from a good water drinking regimen:

- It aids in digestion. A sufficient amount of water helps to breakdown food.
- It nourishes skin. Skins cells like all other cells are made up with water and will not function without it.
- It helps increase memory. Mild dehydration can reduce your mental energy and capacity causing memory to be impaired.
- Carries nutrients and oxygen to your body cells and keeps everything moving.
- It reduces fatigue caused by dehydration.
- It removes toxins from your body. Water is a natural lubricant that softens stool and promotes evacuation of the bowels and reduces the possibility of constipation.
- It regulates your body's cooling system and temperature.
- It aids in circulation and helps to better circulate blood.
- It reduces the risk of colon and bladder cancer.
- It helps to lubricate joints. The lining of the cartilage between the joints use water as a cushion between the bones so that the joints can move easily.

So start right now getting into the habit of drinking water. Start and end each day with a glass of water and make sure to drink at least 2 glasses before lunch. Then have one with lunch, 2 before supper, and one in mid evening. Don't be afraid to drink a few extra. And, by the way, beer does not count as water.

"The secret to living longer is to walk double, eat half, laugh triple, and love without measure."

(And, of course, drink more water.)

~ 47 ~

Christmas and Other Holidays - A Time for Happiness and Sadness

This post is going to be a bit more personal than most. For me, Christmas has always been a struggle between the joy that comes with the season, and the sadness that comes from memories of those that I have loved and lost.

My Dad died on my 3rd birthday at the age of 34. As a youngster, I struggled with the sadness I felt for my Mom – especially during the holidays. She did such a wonderful job raising 3 children, but always seemed so lonely, especially during this time of year. I lost my brother at age 27, my sister at age 57, and my niece at age 16. Then I lost my wife and childhood sweetheart of 40 years, Jan, at age 57. Each one of these losses took its toll. There were times when I thought I wouldn't recover. But I did – and I'm much stronger because of it.

From what I have read, and a number of conversations I've had with others, it seems that many folks have this same problem of being torn between joy and sadness at this time of year. I have found through the years that the best anecdote for this is to put aside some specific time to focus on those things which make you sad.

Reminisce in your mind about those you have lost, and the good times you spent together. Cry if you can – it'll do you good. When you are finished, smile and feel happy about how lucky you were to have them in your life. Then move on. You owe it to them, and to yourself to be happy!

And then focus on the joys of your current life. For me, it's my wonderful wife, Jean, and her family, my successful children, my incredible grandchildren, and my health. And that's just for starters. When you begin to look at all those things that are providing joy and meaning to you, there's a pretty good chance you will be surprised at how long the list is. If you are one of the many who deal with the balance between sadness and joy in this Christmas season, I sincerely hope this is helpful to you.

"Inhale the future. Exhale the past."

Reducing Your Stress During the Holidays

For some of us, stress can reach a peak during the holidays. But, whether it's the holiday season or not, we need to keep stress under control. A certain amount of stress is good because it gives us the "push" we need. But too much stress can negatively impact your health by creating:

- o Headaches
- o Digestive Problems o Pain
- o Sleeping Problems
- o Chronic Conditions

So how can you manage your stress? Here are a few stress management techniques you can try:

Deep Breathing
This is perhaps the single best thing you can do. It can bring down your blood pressure in minutes. It is particularly effective in helping you to sleep. Here is how to deep breathe:

- Sit comfortably with your back straight. Put one hand on your chest and the other on your stomach.
- Breathe in through your nose. The hand on your stomach should rise. The hand on your chest should move very little.
- Exhale slowly through your mouth, pushing out as much air as you can while contracting your abdominal muscles. The hand on your stomach should move as you exhale, but your other hand should move very little.
- Now breathe in on a count of 4 and out on a count of 4 (2 rounds)
- Now breathe in a bit deeper on a count of 8 and out on a count of 8 (2 rounds).
- Continue to breathe in through your nose and out through your mouth. Try to inhale enough so that your lower abdomen rises and falls. Count slowly as you exhale.

The positive effect of this exercise may really surprise you! It sure surprised me.

Progressive Muscle Relaxation

- Slowly tense the muscles in your right foot, squeezing as tightly as you can. Hold for a count of 10.

- Relax your right foot and focus on the tension flowing away, and the way your foot feels as it becomes limp and loose.
- Stay in the relaxed state for a moment, breathing deeply and slowly.
- When ready, shift to your left foot, and repeat the process following the same sequence.
- Move slowly up through your body contracting and relaxing muscle groups as you go (right calf, left calf, right thigh, left thigh, stomach etc.).

It may take some practice at first, but try not to tense muscles other than those intended.

Guided Imagery
There is a lot of information out there regarding techniques of guided imagery. In a nutshell, it involves imagining yourself in a place you have always wanted to be and taking a slow, guided tour in your mind. Try this out and enjoy your trip. Its secondary value is that it's the cheapest trip you will ever take!

Laughter
As many of you know, I have a long history in the study of laughter and humor and have had several posts on this topic. Suffice it to say that taking time for laughter and smiles goes a long way in dealing with stress. I'll cover many of the techniques in future posts. My book, **Add Humor To Your Life: Add Life To Your Humor,** will show you dozens of ways to bring laughter into your life (hint, hint).

Stretching
Stretching exercises are great for seniors because they will go a long way toward reducing body stiffness. But they also have good effect on stress. Look up "stretching for seniors" and you'll find all sorts of exercises.

Relaxation Techniques
Finding ways to just totally relax your mind and body can go a long way in reducing stress. Take a nap, read a book, write, have a massage, exercise, practice yoga or tai chi, take a hot shower, or try aroma therapy. Anything that helps you just get away from the things that might be causing stress. By the way, a good night's sleep contributes a lot to reducing stress too.

Hope these help and I hope you all have a wonderful holiday season.

"Your mind is a garden. Your thoughts are seeds. You can grow flowers, or you can grow weeds."

The Art of Wandering and Wondering

Years ago I was facilitating a creative thinking session for a team at Kodak, and we had reached a point where they seemed to run out of ideas. I instructed the team to take a long break, to just wander and wonder, and see what new thoughts come to mind. We were at a venue that had a lot of interesting surroundings, and I asked them to carefully observe these surroundings and try to connect them with the problem we were trying to solve. When they returned, there was an amazing influx of new ideas, and it was then that I learned about the power of wandering and wondering.

A big part of staying young is to always maintain and active mind. There are lots of ways to do this, but the one I want to discuss here is to take time each day to wander and wonder. So let's take a look at a few ways you might carry this out. You can either wander physically or mentally, but to be effective you need to try to always do it with a clear mind.

Here are a couple of ways to physically wander (which will also give you some exercise):

- Take your daily walk in an area that is familiar, and see how many things you can observe that you have never noticed before.
- Take a walk in an unfamiliar area like a park, a mall, a town you have never been in. Jot down some of the interesting and different things you observe (either in your mind or on paper).

Wandering mentally is a little easier and a bit less time consuming:

- Wander through a dictionary and pick a few interesting words that trigger ideas in your mind.
- Read a few magazines that are ones you wouldn't normally read, and jot down some thoughts that come to mind.
- Get on your PC, laptop, IPad, smart phone, souped-up crystal radio, or other device and use a search engine (Google, Bing, DuckDuckGo) to search things that come to mind. The amount of information and ideas you get will amaze you!
- ☐ Search "Old Ads" on the internet and reflect on what impact they had on your life. I have a pretty good collection of these which you can find on my Pinterest site at pinterest.com/lindsayecollier/

Put your own spin on this, and find a few of your own ways to wander and wonder. Have fun with it and do it as often as you can. I'd love to hear your experiences too.

"All who wander are not lost."

George Carlin on Aging

George Carlin was a very funny and brilliant guy (albeit a little raw at times). His take on aging is wonderful, so I thought I'd share some of his thoughts with you. I remember one of his routines which was all about how we define our age at different stages in our lives. It went something like this:

- When you are less than ten years old you think in fractions. "I'm four and a half going on five."

- When you are in your teens you jump to the next number (I'm almost 16). And there is always a ceremony at 21!

- You become 21, turn 30, push 40, reach 50, make it to 60 and hit 70.

- Then it's a day by day thing (I'm still above ground today).

- And when you reach your 90's, you start going backwards (I was just 92).

- And when you reach 100, you become a kid all over again and think in terms of fractions (I'm 100 and a half)

Brilliant, isn't it?

Here are George Carlin's tips for staying young:

1. Throw out nonessential numbers. This includes age, weight and height. Let the doctors worry about them. That is why you pay them.

2. Keep only cheerful friends. The grouches pull you down.

3. Keep learning. Learn more about the computer, crafts, gardening, whatever, even ham radio. Never let the brain idle. 'An idle mind is the devil's workshop.' And the devil's family name is Alzheimer's.

4. Enjoy the simple things.

5. Laugh often, long, and loud. Laugh until you gasp for breath.

6. The tears happen. Endure, grieve, and move on. The only person, who is with us our entire life, is ourselves. Be ALIVE while you are alive.

7. Surround yourself with what you love, whether it's family, pets, keepsakes, music, plants, hobbies, whatever. Your home is your refuge.

8. Cherish your health: If it is good, preserve it. If it is unstable, improve it. If it is beyond what you can improve, get help.

9. Don't take guilt trips. Take a trip to the mall, even to the next county; to a foreign country, but NOT to where the guilt is.

10. Tell the people you love that you love them, at every opportunity.

AND, ALWAYS REMEMBER:

*"Life's journey is not to
arrive at the grave safely
in a well preserved body,
but rather to skid in sideways,
totally used up and worn out, shouting Wo'hoo,
'Man, what a ride"!*

Pinterest - A Great Tool for Tracking Your Life Interests

For several years I have been rather fascinated with Pinterest which is a social media website that allows users to pin and organize images and videos found on the web. So what's this got to do with "growing young"? Through the years we all amass a lot of interests, and this provides a wonderful way of categorizing and sharing these – and adding to them. It's a great way of reliving, and expanding your life interests, and adding excitement to your life.

It's easy, fun, and free – and quite addictive. You begin by creating "boards" that represent your major areas of interest, and then "pinning" things you find to these boards. It's like having a giant corkboard that can be manipulated in countless ways. The material you pin can come from things you find on websites, or from your own material (such as photos). On most every website page you will see the small Pinterest logo which allows you to easily pin it to one of your boards. Boards and pins are easily changed, deleted, or moved.

Click on this logo and it will take you right to your Pinterest site and give you the option of what board you want to pin it to (including a new board).

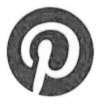

What might you track with Pinterest?

- Cool Products (a special interest of mine)
- Photographs (save your best here)
- Health Issues (save what keeps you healthy)
- Recipes (this is my most used cook book)
- Funny Stuff (cartoons, funny videos, anything that makes you laugh)
- Quotations (one of my favorites)
- Books (show your favorites)
- Creative Ideas You Have (track them or lose them)
- Pet Pictures (tons of these are available)
- Gardening Ideas (a great place to get creative)
- And On and On

There is no limit to how many boards you can have, or how much you can pin to them. And the categories are only limited by your own imagination!

Another thing that comes in handy is that you can make your boards secret so only you can see them. Sometimes you just don't want to share this stuff with anyone. Often I will keep a board that's in the development process secret until it's complete.

Check out my Pinterest site below just to get a few ideas. You may even find some things there that you'll want to pin to your own boards – have at it! That's the beauty of Pinterest. You can greatly expand your interests by copying what others have found in each category. And, as you re -pin from other user's boards, Pinterest will begin sending you more ideas for your own boards. For example, I have always been a follower of great quotes. It turns out that there are a lot of folks on Pinterest with the same interest, and I have been able to add tremendously to my collection. One of my other interests is the tracking of innovative products and gadgets and you will find a lot of these here along with direct links to sources. Check out my site and re-pin to our heart's content.

pinterest.com/lindsayecollier

Give Pinterest a try. You have nothing to lose, and may just find that it will bring some joy and excitement to your life. Enjoy!

"Anyone who keeps the ability to see beauty never grows old."

Franz Kafka

I Love Smoothies

A while back my wife, Jean, bought me a Magic NutriBullet for Christmas. I absolutely love this product! It is well-built, reasonably priced, and lots of fun. More importantly, it makes it so easy to get in the habit of making smoothies for breakfast, lunch, snacks and more. The results are almost always delicious, healthy, and highly nutritious (and surprisingly filling as well). And the possibilities are endless regarding what you can include in them. Of course, any blender will do as well.

My normal smoothie consists of a combination of bananas, strawberries, blueberries, pineapples, apples, and oranges. It's a great way to use up those over ripened bananas too – they taste just as good as fresh ones in the smoothies. Fresh or frozen is okay (but I usually use a couple of frozen fruits which makes the results nicely chilled). I also add protein powder to give it a boost. I add milk and then throw in a little vanilla flavored Coffee Mate which gives it a little extra taste. Some leafy green vegetables are also good.

Also, there are tons of Smoothie cookbooks, many of which are free in their Kindle form. But it's so much fun experimenting with different combinations of ingredients. I can think of maybe only once or twice that an experiment of mine went bad. But, I lived through it!

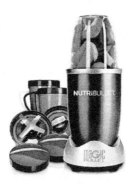

Here's to "Smoothie Sailing"!

"People who are always raising the roof usually don't have much in the attic."

Why Your Sense of Humor Is So Important To You

We all have an absolutely wonderful resource available to us that can have a major influence on our lives. That resource is the ability to access our sense of humor – something we always have at our disposal. There are some 206 bones in the human body, and that's not counting the most important one - the *funny bone*. We all have one, but some of us can't seem to find it. Some people find it easy to use their sense of humor – and some don't.

Humor can make your life more exciting, more satisfying, more vibrant, and, perhaps even longer.

- What part does humor play in your life?
- Do you wake up with a smile on your face?
- How often do you laugh and smile during the day?
- Would you describe yourself as having a sense of humor?
- Do others think you have a sense of humor?
- Are you able to put a humorous spin on things that might appear at first to be serious?
- If you are still working, do you think of "fun work" as an oxymoron?

It's been said that *"Laughter is like changing a diaper. It may not make a permanent difference but it sure improves things for a while"*. This is kind of funny – but it's also dead wrong! Laughter can definitely create a permanent change!

I've been fascinated with humor as a resource for a long time. As a creative thinking and innovation expert in a major corporation, I facilitated hundreds of ideation sessions, and there is one thing I can say for sure. There was always a direct and positive relationship between the amount of laughter and the quality of the thinking derived from these sessions. At one point, I even built what may have been the first corporate *humor room* to help people bring more humor into the workplace.

So why is humor so important in your lives?

It can make you a healthier person by:

- Strengthening your immune system
- Reducing pain – triggering endorphins
- Relaxing and toning muscles (including facial)
- Reducing the effects of stress
- Stimulating digestion and circulation (some think of as an internal organ massage)
- Reducing blood pressure
- Building up facial and throat muscles – reducing snoring
- Cleansing the lungs – like deep breathing, sending more enriched oxygen to the body
- Burning calories

It can strengthen you mentally and emotionally by:

- Helping to dissolve anger and unite people
- Helping us deal with loss and grief
- Helping us cope with change
- Stabilizing mood swings
- Increasing your attention span

It makes you a more interesting person by:

- Attracting others with your smile
- Helping to strengthen your relationships
- Making you more attractive
- Helping us communicate with people from other environments
- Improving your morale
- Enhancing romance
- Improving your outlook on life

It stimulates your thinking process by:

- Stimulating creative thinking
- Helping the learning process
- Helping us get our message across
- Helping us remember

If you really want the scoop on humor in your life, check out the best book ever on the topic (It really is -I'm not just saying that because I wrote the book). I hope you are okay with my shameless book plugs. Remember, I am just doing this to make you a happy right up through your golden years, and this book is guaranteed to do that. Go to Amamzon.com and enter, 'Add Humor to Your Life'.

"A person without a sense of humor is like a wagon without springs –
jolted by every pebble on the road."

Henry Ward Beecher

How to Awaken the Child Within

One of my favorites quotations is "**It's never too late to have a happy childhood.**" Here is some sage advice I found in my archives on how to bring out that inner child in you.

Do you remember how wonderfully carefree you were as a child? Children are typically honest, innocent sources of steady outpourings of love. They are naturally curious and ask questions, and they are mystified by objects and experiences we have long since chosen to take for granted. I certainly miss that outlook on life and every once in a while, letting a childlike mentality take control is exactly the springboard I need to help me feel refreshed.

Jump back into those adorably small, yet ridiculously patterned outfits, and let your inner child emerge once again.

Believe in miracles.

In a world where research is the basis for drawing conclusions and reason is rewarded, allow yourself to believe the unbelievable in life. The word itself, *miracle*, often seems magical or childish. But don't let the unexplainable just slip by without at least a nod of recognition. Believing in miracles allows these experiences to be much more valuable. Help them along by allowing your imagination to get involved.

Jump for joy.

Today, getting excited may involve a gasp or a fist-pump (or maybe no reaction at all). But remember when you literally *jumped for joy*? We should learn to employ that vigorous enthusiasm to our lives a bit more often. And if you find the act of jumping too embarrassing (a very adult outlook), then at least allow your soul to jump for joy. Do something that you know will give you that sensation of happiness. I'm sure you won't regret it.

Get Silly.

Nourish your inner child by being completely silly with friends or by enjoying an activity you wouldn't normally do. Taking that step to simply play and expend energy will produce a newfound sense of awe. The feeling of wonder that comes with peeling back the layers of thought and assessment is lost all too often in adulthood. With that in mind, play before you give it a second thought, and let the thrill of life take over.

Draw outside the lines.

It seems so simple, but we spend our days caged in by boundaries and consequences. While these concepts define our comfort zone, sometimes tearing down those walls and exposing our imperfections takes us to a place of greater learning. A child's uninhibited attitude toward tasks and challenges is admirable, and certainly something to learn from.

Love unconditionally.

Why do we tie strings to our love? And when did we learn to do that? One of the most beautiful things about children is their ability to love. They love unconditionally their families, their neighbors, their everyday experiences, and people from all walks of life-they love questioning the world itself! It's amazing (and disappointing) that we can lose this ability as we grow. Reclaim your ability to love unconditionally-even if it's just for an hour.

I hope that some of these tips bring back old memories and attitudes that you're willing to rely on once more. It's amazing how simple and positive a child's outlook is. I suppose that with time and experience, our perspective becomes convoluted and much less naive (with both positive and negative influences). Nevertheless, relish your inner child, and enjoy the simplicity and beauty of living all over again.

Have a happy childhood and keep growing young!

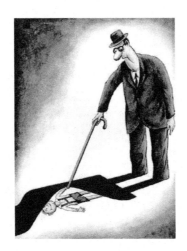

"The older *you* get, the more important it is not to act your age."

Inspiration through Quotations

I have been a quotations nut for many, many years. The way I figure it, there are a lot of people who are a lot smarter than me and, if I can learn from them, I'll be better off. I began collecting quotes during my years as an expert in creative thinking, and most of them focused on that topic. One of my first books (Quotations to Tickle Your Brain) was a compilation of this collection.

Now that I am in my "mature" years, I am much more interested in quotes that leave powerful messages about life, particularly the life of us seniors. I want to share some of the most meaningful ones with you but, to be honest, I'm not sure where to begin since I have so many. You can see what I'm talking about if you visit my quotes board on my Pinterest page. Feel free to copy and paste any of these that are particularly interesting to you.

So I think I will throw a dart at my quotes board, and find a few that may pique your interest. Here goes!

"Worrying is like sitting in a rocking chair. It gives you something to do but doesn't get you anywhere."

What would your life be like if you didn't worry about a thing? When is the last time you decided not to try something because you were worried that you'd fail? What are some things you can do to keep you from worrying? Play with this in your mind for a while and see what happens.

"Don't worry about getting old, worry about thinking old."

This speaks so well to the purpose of this book which is all about "thinking young". Earle Nightingale's secret to life is *"You are what you think"*. So one thing you should stop worrying about is getting old. You can't change that, but your journey will be so much better if you spend these years "thinking young". The more you can think of yourself as young, the easier it will be to grow young.

"How others see you is not important. How you see yourself means everything!"

How would things be different for you if you weren't quite so concerned about how others saw you, and focused on raising how you see yourself to a new level? I think a lot of us who are over fifty (in my case, way over) begin to think of ourselves as less adequate. After all, we have likely achieved most of our goals, and perhaps lost some of the driving force that has kept us going through the years. It might be time to reestablish some new goals, and maybe even bring the child in you back.

"You are never too old to set another goal or dream another dream."

When we were younger our lives were full of dreams and goals. Hopefully you have achieved all of these, but just because you are older, doesn't mean you have to stop dreaming of things you would like to explore, achieve, and do. So begin setting some new goals for your future now.

"Aging is an extraordinary process where you become the person you always should have."

This is a quotation from David Bowie no less (many of the rock and pop stars really do have brains). Sometimes it takes years to learn some of the more meaningful lessons of life. What are some of the basic lessons you have learned through the years? How might you put these lessons to good use in your next 50 years? In a nutshell, try to take David Bowie's advice and work on becoming the person you always should have been."

"Life would be infinitely happier if we could be born at eighty and gradually approach eighteen."

Mark Twain

How would you be living your life if you were actually working your way back to 18 years old? What would you be doing differently? What's keeping you from living as if you are really growing younger? So, just go with it!

I've just scratched the surface with this and have a lot more inspirational quotes to share. Stay tuned.

"Expecting things to change without putting in any effort is like waiting for a ship at an airport."

The Story of the Stonecutter

Fables and stories can serve as great lessons of life, and this Chinese folk tale, *The Story of the Stonecutter* (from The Tao of Pooh), has some very powerful lessons. Read it over a couple of times and ask yourself how it may relate to your own life experiences. This may require a bit of deep thinking, but I promise you it won't hurt a bit – and you just may come out with some interesting revelations!

"There was once a stonecutter who was dissatisfied with himself and with his position in life.

One day he passed a wealthy merchant's house. Through the open gateway, he saw many fine possessions and important visitors. "How powerful that merchant must be!" thought the stonecutter. He became very envious and wished that he could be like the merchant.

To his great surprise, he suddenly became the merchant, enjoying more luxuries and power than he had ever imagined, but envied and detested by those less wealthy than himself. Soon a high official passed by, carried in a sedan chair, accompanied by attendants and escorted by soldiers beating gongs. Everyone, no matter how wealthy, had to bow low before the procession. "How powerful that official is!" he thought. "I wish that I could be a high official!"

Then he became the high official, carried everywhere in his embroidered sedan chair, feared and hated by the people all around. It was a hot summer day, so the official felt very uncomfortable in the sticky sedan chair. He looked up at the sun. It shone proudly in the sky, unaffected by his presence. "How powerful the sun is!" he thought. "I wish that I could be the sun!"

Then he became the sun, shining fiercely down on everyone, scorching the fields, cursed by the farmers and laborers. But a huge black cloud moved between him and the earth, so that his light could no longer shine on everything below. "How powerful that storm cloud is!" he thought. "I wish that I could be a cloud!"

Then he became the cloud, flooding the fields and villages, shouted at by everyone. But soon he found that he was being pushed away by some great force, and realized that it was the wind. "How powerful it is!" he thought. "I wish that I could be the wind!"
Then he became the wind, blowing tiles off the roofs of houses, uprooting trees, feared and hated by all below him. But after a while, he ran up

against something that would not move, no matter how forcefully he blew against it – a huge, towering rock. "How powerful that rock is!" he thought. "I wish that I could be a rock!"

Then he became the rock, more powerful than anything else on earth. But as he stood there, he heard the sound of a hammer pounding a chisel into the hard surface, and felt himself being changed. "What could be more powerful than I, the rock?" he thought.

He looked down and saw far below him the figure of a stonecutter."

You are probably thinking that was interesting, but don't leave yet. Read it over again and do a bit of deep thinking as to its possible meaning for you. Enjoy the experience!

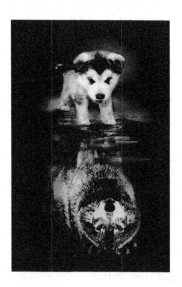

"The road to success is always under construction."

Health Benefits of Asparagus

Asparagus has so many health benefits; it should be added to the every healthy diet. Asparagus is great as a detox vegetable, an **anti-aging vegetable,** an aphrodisiac, and much more. Based on my experience, people either love this veggie, or hate it. There seems to be no in between. I'm on the love side myself. And it's so easy to prepare. The two easiest ways I've found are to either sauté it in olive oil until crisp, or just wrap it in a paper towel and microwave it for 1 ½ - 2 minutes.

Asparagus is a member of the lily family. It grows easily in the home garden right in the flower bed – it is a perennial and can yield a harvest for decades. Asparagus can be planted as seeds or roots any time of the year.

Here is a list of some of the health benefits of asparagus followed by a list further explaining those health benefits.

Detoxifies

Asparagus has 288 milligrams of potassium per cup. Potassium is known for reducing belly fat. It also contains 3 grams of fiber which cleanses the digestive system. It has virtually no natural sodium, has no fat or cholesterol, and one cup has only 40 calories. According to a clinical dietician at UCLA Medical Center, asparagus in the ultimate in detox vegetables.

Has Anti-Aging functions

Asparagus is rich in potassium, vitamin A, and folate. It is also very high in glutathione – an amino acid compound with potent antioxidant properties; a must as an anti-aging deterrent. Glutathione (GSH) is an antioxidant that protects cells from toxins such as free radicals.

Can protect against cancer

Folate is now known to be an important protection against cancer and, as we've seen, asparagus has a high concentrate of this.

Reducing the risk of heart disease

Heart disease is one thing I have had to deal with in my own life. Fortunately things are well under control. Folic Acid supplements are often recommended for this, but eating whole foods like asparagus in a much better option.

Can prevent osteoporosis and arthritis

Asparagus has vitamin K which studies have shown can help prevent osteoporosis and osteoarthritis. Vitamin K aids in bone formation and repair. It is also necessary for the synthesis of osteocalcin. Osteocalcin is the protein in bone tissue on which calcium crystallizes. Asparagus has been listed as the number one source of vitamin K.

<ins>Is considered an aphrodisiac</ins>

Asparagus is considered a psycho-physiological aphrodisiac because of its shape. It is said to trigger the mind to have a physiological response. The French word for asparagus is asperge; asperge is a slang word for penis.

Reduces pain and inflammation

This is another benefit of the folate contained in this veggie.

Additionally, studies have shown that the nutritional benefits of asparagus can help prevent and treat urinary tract infections and kidney stones. Overall, asparagus is rich in potassium, vitamin A, folate, glutathione, and vitamin K. It is high in fiber, has no sodium, is low in calories and has no cholesterol or fat.

If you're one of those who say you hate asparagus, there are a lot of reasons to get to like it. There are also a lots of delicious asparagus recipes. Just look them up on the net.

"You must be willing to lose the way, to find the way."

Your Smile Is Your Biggest Asset

Smiling is just a mild form of laughter, but it's a great beginning. As they say,"A smile changes your face value". Begin each day with a smile, even if you have to force yourself into it. Get up, look yourself in the mirror, and flash the biggest, silliest, stupidest grin you can come up with. Then raise this smile to a new, higher level till the corners of your mouth nearly meet your ear lobes. You might want to make sure nobody is watching you, or they might take steps to have you committed. If you feel down during the day for some reason, then repeat this process if you can.

Try to carry your smile with you all day. That doesn't mean you need to be constantly smiling, but it does mean you need to be ready to smile at all times. Incidentally, if you have difficulty perfecting your smile, you may want begin by using a *smile stick*. You can order these at smilestick.com for just a few bucks. Keep some in your home, office, car, or wherever you think might be appropriate.

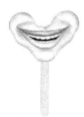

For years while I was driving back and forth to work, I would carry a *smile stick* in my car, and I found a number of opportunities to put it to good use. For example, if I pulled up to one of those people who looked like death-warmed-over on their way to work, I would flash them a big grin with my smile stick. I think in some cases it made their day – and it also helped me to start mine on a positive, happy note.

Smile at everyone you encounter. Never miss the opportunity to smile at someone you meet, or just pass by. You don't always need the ear to ear smile – just a pleasant smile that says you are glad to see them may suffice. A nice greeting along with it is always welcome too. You'll feel good and they probably will too.

Always look for an opportunity to share some laughter with the people you meet. If something tickles your funny bone don't hesitate in sharing this with those around you, even if they are total strangers. And never bypass an opportunity to laugh (with gusto if possible) when someone shares something with you that they think is funny. If it isn't that funny then just fake it a bit.

If you need something that will really put a big smile on your face and a lot of laughter in your soul, check out my book, ***The Funniest Book You Will Ever Read. Period!*** This book is a compilation of my collection of funny stuff over the past several decades, and is just full of some of the funniest things you will ever see. I think I may just have made another shameless plug – sorry.

And don't forget to give yourself a big smile in the mirror every evening before you go to bed. I guarantee you'll get a better night's sleep!

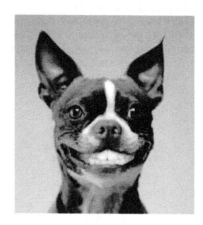

"Smiling is the second best thing you can do with your lips."

A Few Snippets from My 'Silly File'

In my books and presentations, I often suggest that you keep a "Silly File" or two. I keep a digital file on Microsoft Word as well as a hard copy file in a manila folder in my file cabinet. I refer to them often when I need some material or just some cheering up. Here are just a few items from my *Silly File*.

The man and wife at the dentist

A man and his wife walked into a dentist's office. The man said to the dentist, "Doc, I'm in one heck of a hurry. I have two buddies sitting out in my car waiting for us to go play golf, so forget about the anesthetic, I don't have time for the gums to get numb. I just want you to pull the tooth, and be done with it! We have a 10:00 AM tee time at the best golf course in town and it's 9:30 already. I don't have time to wait for the anesthetic to work!'
The dentist thought to himself, "My goodness, this is surely a very brave man asking to have his tooth pulled without using anything to kill the pain." So the dentist asks him, "Which tooth is it sir?"The man turned to his wife and said, "Open your mouth, Honey, and show him."

The Florida senior citizen

A Florida senior citizen drove his brand new Corvette convertible out of the dealership. Taking off down the road, he pushed it to 80 mph, enjoying the wind blowing through what little hair he had left. "Amazing," he thought as he flew down I-95, pushing the pedal even more.

Looking in his rear view mirror, he saw a Florida State Trooper, blue lights flashing, and siren blaring. He floored it to 100 mph, then 110, then 120. Suddenly he thought, "What am I doing? I'm too old for this!" and pulled over to await the trooper's arrival.

Pulling in behind him, the trooper got out of his vehicle and walked up to the Corvette. He looked at his watch, then said, "Sir, my shift ends in 30 minutes. Today is Friday. If you can give me a new reason for speeding – a reason I've never before heard – I'll let you go."

The old gentleman paused then said, "Three years ago, my wife ran off with a Florida State Trooper. I thought you were bringing her back. "Have a good day, Sir," replied the trooper.

Old couple getting married

Jacob, age 92, and **Mary**, age 89, living in The Villages, are all excited about their decision to get married. They go for a stroll to discuss the wedding, and on the way they pa.. drugstore. Jacob suggests they go in. Jacob addresses the man behind the counter:

"Are you the owner?" The pharmacist answers, "Yes."

Jacob: "We're about to get married. Do you sell heart medication?"
Pharmacist: "Of course we do."
Jacob: "How about medicine for circulation?"
Pharmacist: "All kinds."
Jacob: "Medicine for rheumatism?"
Pharmacist: "Definitely."
Jacob: "How about suppositories and medicine for impotence?"
Pharmacist: "You bet!"
Jacob: "Medicine for memory problems, arthritis and Alzheimer's?"
Pharmacist: "Yes, a large variety. The works."
Jacob: "What about vitamins, sleeping pills, Geritol, antidotes for Parkinson's disease?"
Pharmacist: "Absolutely."
Jacob: "Everything for heartburn and indigestion?"

Pharmacist: "We sure do."
Jacob: "You sell wheelchairs and walkers and canes?"
Pharmacist: "All speeds and sizes."
Jacob: "Adult diapers?"
Pharmacist: "Sure."
Jacob: "We'd like to use this store as our Bridal Registry."

Cigar Insurance

Here is a short article I saw in the paper a while back:

Without honesty, karma has a funny way of catching up. Consider the cigar smoker who purchased several hundred expensive stogies and had them insured against fire. After he smoked them, he filed a claim pointing out that they had indeed been destroyed by fire.

The insurance company refused to pay, so the man sued. The judge ruled in the man's favor saying that the cigars had indeed been insured against, and been destroyed by fire. So the insurance company paid the claim and, when the man accepted the money, promptly had him arrested for arson.

"Life is short. Smile while you still have teeth."

Do Something Dumb or Silly Each Day

We need to reserve some time for doing things that have perhaps no redeeming value whatsoever other than to take us away from reality for a spell. If you like to spend time on your computer you may want to cruise around sites like _dumb.com_. This site offers a plethora of dumb things to do including dumb facts, chatting with God, old time radio, funny bumper stickers, a virtual Voodoo doll to torture your friends, and even a virtual bubble wrap that could entertain you for hours. There are over 100 things to see and do here. Go there right now!

Or you could just _google_ around using words like dumb, silly, stupid etc. You'll be amazed at what you find. If reading is your thing, go pick up some marginally useless books generally found in the humor section. Take some time away from "War and Peace" to peruse these dumb books.

Ones I particularly like are cartoons like _The Far Side_ and _Quigmans_. _The Book of Stupid Questions_ by Tom Weller also comes to mind as does the _Imponderables Collection_ of David Feldman (Why Do Clocks Run Clockwise?) And any book by David Barry is worth keeping around for those times when you really need to get the cobwebs out of your head. His best are _Babies and Other Hazards of Sex, Stay Fit and Healthy Until You're Dead_, and _Claw Your Way to the Top of the Organization_ . For visual stimulation of dumb stuff there is nothing better than reruns of _Monty Python's Flying Circus_.

You also might want to take some time to just do dumb things as well such as:

- Call Dial-A-Prayer and argue with them.
- Walk or drive backwards through a drive-up window.
- Grow a beard (men only please) that will undoubtedly make you look older (ala Santa Claus). Then shave it off to take years off your life.
- Get a coloring book and have at it.
- Have a serious conversation with your dog or cat (or your neighbor's pet if you don't have one of your own).
- Try "doodling". I know I'm dating myself but there was a time when doodling was the rage. It involves drawing what comes to mind. Get a pencil and a sketch pad and let your thoughts flow.
- ☐ Wander around YouTube. You'd be amazed at how much is there and a lot of it is really dumb.

I wouldn't classify this as dumb stuff, but I find that just spending time listening to some music (without anything else going on) can be very stimulating. I like almost all forms of music but especially classical and jazz. Find a comfortable chair, put on the earphones and just immerse yourself in some great piece of music for a while and see what happens.

I could go on and on here because I've done a lot of marginally dumb things in my life. Quite a few years ago I wrote a book called **Get Out of Your Thinking Box; 365 Ways To Brighten Your Life and Enhance Your Creativity**. In it you will find a whole pile of things to do to tweak your thinking and tickle your funny bone. Here are a few items from this book:

- Call a random number and just wish someone a nice day.
- Look at the world as if your eyes were on your knee caps.
- Have a "whine and Jeez" party.
- Come up with a nonsense language and use it with your friends.
- Listen to some old time radio shows (dumb.com).
- Go to a bank and ask for change for a nickel.
- Think of all the ways your life is like a *slinky*.
- Go skip rocks on a pond.
- Go test drive an 18 wheeler.
- Wear a silly hat all day.
- Spell check all your friends names and see what comes up. One of my friends' names came up as "cheery hormones".
- Interview some people telling them you are writing a book on some strange topic.
- Carry out a conversation with someone as if you are an opera singer.
- Pretend you are a sponge for a day and soak up everything you can. Wring yourself out at the end of the day. If your name is 'Bob" skip this one.
- Tap dance.
- Write down all the things that are bothering you on a roll of toilet paper – and flush it.
- Try your best to be dyslexic for a day.
- Think of some things that you've never thought about before.
- Visit a cemetery and read the epitaphs.
- Create your own personal logo.
- Try to have a serious conversation with your dog or cat.
- Build a house of cards.
- Think of as many stupid questions as you can (even though there is no such thing as a stupid question).
- Browse through a library.
- Read a Dr. Seuss book.
- View the world from the perspective of an insect.

At some point you may want to get back to reality. Have fun with this and take your significant other on this trip if you can.

"If you don't live on the edge sometimes, you will never see the view."

Reliving Your Memories

I was inspired to write this short article when I came across a Facebook post that said, "Without saying your age, what are some of the things from your childhood you remember that a younger person would not understand?" It caused me to take a trip down my own memory lane and, I must admit, it was a very pleasant journey. Jot down some of your answers to this question.

So, what can you do to stimulate some thoughts as to these memories? Start by going to ThePeoplesHistory.com and check out what was happening when you were born. I think you'll find this pretty interesting. Then check out what was happening at various key years in your life (school graduations, family milestones, work life milestones, etc.). Try to remember what life was like in those periods, and spend a little time reliving these in your mind.

Google "old ads" and take a look at some of these that may have particular meaning for you. Check out vintageads.com and check on the years that were important to you. Reflect on these and try to relive memories associated with them. Here are three ads I picked at random from my Pinterest page (I have a pretty big collection on my Old Adds board there).

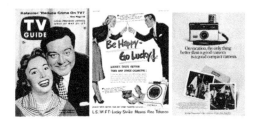

What were you doing and thinking when these ads came out? What memories do they bring to mind? Do they bring out some smiles?

A fun trip through some old comedy routines always brings back a lot of memories. So many of these are available on YouTube and all you have to do is go o YouTube.com and search for a one of your favorite comedians. Also take a trip through some old TV or radio programs and old movies (Young Frankenstein and Blazing Saddles come to mind) on YouTube. Have some fun with this and take these trips often to relive your memories. You'll feel younger when you do this! Enjoy!

"No one is remembered for being normal."

Albert Einstein

Using 'Trim Tabs' in Your Life

Trim tabs are small surfaces connected to the trailing edge of a larger control surface on a boat or aircraft, used to control the trim of the controls, i.e. to counteract hydro- or aerodynamic forces and stabilize the boat or aircraft in a particular desired attitude without the need for the operator to constantly apply a control force. This is done by adjusting the angle of the tab relative to the larger surface.

Buckminster Fuller, one of the great geniuses of the 20th century, loved the metaphor of "trim tabs" for understanding how to leverage personal power. "Bucky" was famous for inventing the *geodesic dome,* and coining the word 'synergy'. After experiencing some rather challenging events in his life an interesting thought came to him:

"Something hit me very hard once, thinking about what one little man could do. Think of the Queen Mary — the whole ship goes by and then comes the rudder. And there's a tiny thing at the edge of the rudder called a trim tab. It's a miniature rudder. Just moving the little trim tab builds a low pressure that pulls the rudder around. It takes almost no effort at all. So I said that the little individual can be a trim tab that could give the power to one person to affect society"

Why not think of the power of the trim tab metaphor in a more personal way? Instead of trying to change society, what about the changes it could make in your life? What personal *trim tabs* could you find to create small shifts in your awareness or behavior that might leverage a much larger effect in your life? How might the idea of trim tabs affect your life?

When I think about trim tabs, the first thing that pops into my mind is how something very small can have such a huge influence on something very massive. A relatively tiny *trim tab* will help to easily turn a large rudder which will in turn change the course of a massive ship or aircraft. Are there some things you can change in your life using one of your small *trim tabs*? Here are a few possibilities. Feel free to add some of your own.

Do small favors for your family and friends. You don't have to paint your neighbors house or anything like that. Just keep an eye out for opportunities to help people out in ways that show you care. The reward to you could be some substantial positive changes in your relationships.

Don't hesitate to thank people, and show your gratitude. Just the words, "Thanks. I appreciate it", can create a very positive change in how people feel about you.

Appreciate every moment of your life – even the small ones. Let the things you enjoy, no matter how small they seem, serve as *trim tabs* to steer you in the right direction.

Try to look at things you 'have to' do in a different way. Learn how to look forward to them instead, and convince yourself that they are things that you 'get to do' rather than 'have to do'. That mental shift becomes a *trim tab* for change. You will begin feeling that you are lucky to be able to do anything in your life, even those things that you have been resisting. The more you can appreciate each moment in your life, the happier you will be.

Spend some time thinking about how some other *trim tabs* in your life can help you move forward in some exciting directions. And have some fun in the process.

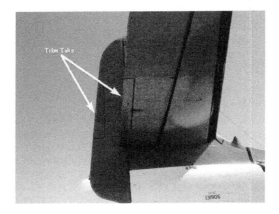

"There is a fountain of youth: It's in your mind, your talents, and the creativity you bring to life and the lives of people you love. When you learn to tap this source, you will truly have defeated age."

Sophia Loren

Seven Steps to Longevity

A while back I attended a talk by a nutritionist (whose name I have sadly forgotten) titled, 'Seven Steps to Longevity'. As many of you know (especially those who have read **_How To Live Happily Ever After_**), I have a lot of interesting views of my own on this topic. He was a very good speaker and, in a nutshell, here are the seven steps he shared:

1. Stay active and mobile
2. Be able To adapt to loss
3. Be socially connected
4. Belong To a faith based community
5. Watch your weight
6. Reduce cardiovascular threat
7. Have a close personal friend and confident

These are pretty close to some of the ones in my book which contains 12 things to do to live forever-guaranteed!

But he spent a long time discussing the last one which he said was so important that, not having it was worse for your health than smoking! This thought has stuck in my mind because, to be quite honest, I think I may actually fall into the category of not having a close confidant. I have many friends, neighbors, associates, a loving wife, children and grandchildren who I love and treasure. But I have difficulty confiding in any of them about my innermost feelings. I blame myself more than I do them for this, and my goal is to reach out more in the near future.

If you have no one with which to share your innermost thoughts, you will be internalizing them, and it just makes sense that this will eventually erode your ability to be happy. Do you have a close personal friend and confidant? If the answer to this is 'no' then you, like me, should be searching for one. It may help you clear out a lot of baggage that is preventing you from attaining real happiness.

Good luck!

"Happiness is like a butterfly. The more you chase it, the more it will elude you. But if you turn your attention to other things, it will come and sit softly on your shoulder."

The Train of Life

A while back a friend sent me an email that I just feel I need to pass on. As I've said before, I love metaphors and use them all the time in my thinking, writing and conversation. This one provides a great learning experience for your life. Enjoy it, and pass it on to those you care about. You can also find it easily on YouTube.

At birth we board a train and meet our parents. We believe they will always travel by our side. However, at some station, our parents will step down from the train, leaving us on this journey alone.

As time goes by, other people will board the train, and they will be significant – siblings, friends, the love of your life, children, and many others. Some will step down and leave a permanent vacuum. Others will go so unnoticed that we won't realize they vacated their seats. The train ride will be full of joy, sorrow, fantasy, expectations, hellos, good-byes, and farewells. A successful ride requires having a good relationship with all passengers. We must give the best of ourselves.

The mystery to everyone is, we do not know at which station we ourselves will step down. So, we must live in the best way, love, forgive, and offer the best of who we are. It is important to do this because when the time comes for us to step down and leave our seat empty we should leave behind beautiful memories for those who will continue to travel on the train of life. I wish you a joyful journey on the train of life. Reap success and give lots of love. More importantly, thank God for the journey.

Lastly, I thank you for being one of the passengers on my train.

What more can I say about this? Nice, isn't it?

"When life knocks you down, rollover and look at the stars."

Some of the Funniest People I Have Ever Known

Humor has always been a big part of my life and I hope it's a big part of yours too. If not, you need to work on that. You'll find a number of posts about humor in this book. But now it's time for a humor break. Here are just a few of the funniest people I've known in my lifetime.

Dave Barry

Dave Barry was a syndicated columnist for the Miami Herald until 2005, and has written a whole bunch of books. These are my all-time favorite humor books, and perhaps the only ones which will make me laugh out loud while alone. You absolutely need to have a few of his books in your library! Here are some of my favorites:

- Babies and Other Hazards of Sex
- Homes and Other Black Holes
- Stay Fit and Healthy, Until You're Dead
- Claw Your Way to the Top: How to Become the Head of a Corporation in Roughly a Week
- Dave Barry's Greatest Hits
- Dave Barry Turns 40, and Dave Barry Turns 50

Go to his Amazon author page for the full listing.

Foster Brooks

Foster was best known as the "Lovable Lush" and one of the best "roasters" ever. Here are a few of his best routines. As an aside, we lived near Foster who was in Rush, New York, a suburb of Rochester. I saw him a couple of times at our local Wegman's market but he was stone sober. I waited for him to break into his routine at the checkout but was disappointed.

The Brain Surgeon

The Airline Pilot

Foster Roasts Don Rickles

Cast of Carol Burnett

Why can't anyone put together a show today like *The Carol Burnett Show*? The combination of Carol along with Harvey Korman, Tin Conway, and Vicki Lawrence was absolutely hysterical. Look for some of the" best of" DVD's. Here are a couple of snippets:

Carol Burnett - No Frills Airline

Carol Burnett Show - Old Man in Surgery

Carol Burnett Show Dentist

Bob Hope

Will there ever be someone as funny, and as giving as this guy? Here is an example of some of his great lines.

ON TURNING 70
'I still chase women, but only downhill'.

ON TURNING 80
'That's the time of your life when even your birthday suit needs pressing.'

ON TURNING 90
'You know you're getting old when the candles cost more than the cake.'

ON TURNING 100
'I don't feel old. In fact, I don't feel anything until noon. Then it's time for my nap.'

ON GIVING UP HIS EARLY CAREER, BOXING
'I ruined my hands in the ring. The referee kept stepping on them.'

ON NEVER WINNING AN OSCAR
'Welcome to the Academy Awards or, as it's called at my home, 'Passover'.

ON GOLF
'Golf is my profession. Show business is just to pay the green fees.'

ON PRESIDENTS
'I have performed for 12 presidents and entertained only six.'

ON WHY HE CHOSE SHOWBIZ FOR HIS CAREER
'When I was born, the doctor said to my mother, Congratulations, you have an eight pound ham.

ON RECEIVING THE CONGRESSIONAL GOLD MEDAL
'I feel very humble, but I think I have the strength of character to fight it.'

ON HIS FAMILY'S EARLY POVERTY
'Four of us slept in the one bed. When it got cold, mother threw on another brother.'

ON HIS SIX BROTHERS
'That's how I learned to dance. Waiting for the bathroom.'

ON HIS EARLY FAILURES
'I would not have had anything to eat if it wasn't for the stuff the audience threw at me.'

ON GOING TO HEAVEN
'I've done benefits for ALL religions. I'd hate to blow the hereafter on a technicality.'

YouTube is loaded with examples of Bob Hope but he is probably best loved for his many visits with our troops. See Bob Hope Through The Years With The Troops and you'll see what I'm talking about.

Robin Williams

He was a true comic genius and master of spontaneity – such a terrible loss. Here are a couple of his YouTube's. The golf routine is one of the funniest routines I've ever seen but, warning, it can get a bit crude. There are a number his full routines on YouTube if you have some extra time.

Robin Williams - Golf

Robin Williams as the American Flag

"No matter how talented, rich or intelligent you are, how you treat animals tells me all I need to know about you."

A Look Back At the Whack-A-Mole Theory

Years ago I wrote my first book, **The Whack-A-Mole Theory**, which focused on how organizations can create breakthrough change. I used this carnival game as a metaphor for how organizations tended to spend most of their time "whacking moles" rather than creating their potential futures. For those who are not familiar with this game, you have a large mallet that you use to whack moles as they randomly pop up from holes in a board. It's lots of fun, but when you are finished you are just left with a blank board.

When I thought back on how I used this metaphor for organizational change, it occurred to me that it is also a great metaphor for our own personal lives. Do you spend a good part of your life whacking moles (solving problems) rather than creating new opportunities? I believe the majority of us, if we were completely honest with ourselves, would answer 'yes' to this. How might your life change if you were to spend less time solving problems and more time focusing on new possibilities?

A book that influenced my thought process as I was writing this book was "*The Path of Least Resistance*" by Robert Fritz. In his book he talks about two approaches to life – *reactive and creative*. If you are in the *reactive* mode you are spending your life just reacting to things that come your way. Obviously you have to do this sometime but, if you spend all your time just reacting to things, you never really advance to anything new. In the creative mode, your mindset is focused on things that will allow you to move on to new opportunities.

The key is to find the right balance between *reactive* and *creative*. It's interesting to note that you can move from *reactive* to *creative* by just moving the 'c' to the front.

So what? Do a quick examination of the balance between reactive and creative in your life. If you are heavy on the reactive side, ask yourself how you might move more into creative activities that might help you find new opportunities. And don't ever think that you are too old to create these new possibilities – because you are never too old for this.

"When it comes to the future there are three kinds of people - Those who let it happen, those who make it happen, and those who wonder what happened."

24 Interludes of Life

I am not sure where this came from but it is well worth sharing in its original form.

1. Don't go for looks, they can deceive. Don't go for wealth even that fades away. Go for someone who makes you smile.
2. There are moments in life when you really miss someone and want to pick them up from your dreams and hug them. Hope you dream of that someone.
3. Dream what you want to dream, go where you want to go, be what you want to be, because you have only one life and one chance to do all the things you want in life.
4. May you have:
   Enough happiness to make you sweet
   Enough trials to make you strong
   Enough sorrow to keep you human
   Enough hope to make you happy
   And enough money to buy gifts.
5. When one door of happiness closes, another opens. But we often look so long at the closed door, that we don't see the one which has been opened for us.
6. The best kind of friend is the one you could sit on a porch, swing with, never saying a word and then walk away feeling like that was the best conversation you've had.
7. It's true that we don't know what we've got until we lose it, but it's also true that we don't know what we've been missing until it arrives.
8. Always put yourself in other's shoes. If you feel that it hurts you, it probably hurts them too.
9. A careless word may kindle strife, a cruel word may wreck a life, a timely word may level stress, a lovely word may heal and bless.
10. The beginning of love is to let those we love be perfectly themselves, and not to twist them with our own image. Otherwise we love only the reflection of ourselves we find in them.
11. The happiest people don't necessarily have the best of everything; they just make the most of everything that comes along the way.
12. Maybe God wants us to meet a few wrong people before meeting the right one so that, when we finally meet the right person, we should know how to be grateful for that gift.
13. It takes a minute to have a crush on someone, an hour to like someone and a day to love someone – but it takes a lifetime to forget someone.
14. Happiness lies for those who cry, those who hurt, those who have searched and those who have tried. For only they can appreciate the importance of people who have touched their lives.
15. Love is when you take away the feeling, the passion, the romance and find out you still care for that person.
16. A sad thing about life is that when you meet someone who means a lot to you only to find out in the end that it was never bound to be and you just have to let go.
17. Love starts with a smile, develops with a kiss and ends with a tear.

18. Love comes to those who still hope even though they've been disappointed, to those who still believe even though they've been betrayed

19. It hurts to love someone, and not to be loved in return. But what is most painful is to love someone and never finds the courage to let the person know how you feel.

20. The brightest future will always be based on a forgotten past. You can't go on well in life until you let go of your past failures and heartaches.

21. Never say goodbye when you still want to try. Never give up when you still feel you can take it. Never say you don't love that person anymore when you can't let go.

22. Giving someone all your love is never an assurance that they'll love you back. Don't expect love in return; just wait for it to grow in their hearts. But if it doesn't, be content it grew in yours.

23. There are things you love to hear but you would never hear it from the person whom you would like to hear it from, but don't be deaf to hear it from the person who says it with his heart.

24. When you were born, you were crying and everyone around you was smiling. Live your life to the fullest so that when you die, you're smiling and everyone around you is crying.

I particularly like the last one and have used it often.

"A beautiful face will age and a perfect body will change. But a beautiful soul will always be a beautiful soul."

Time for Some Laughter

For years I have kept track of the things that made me laugh in what I call my "Silly File". I have a hard copy version and a Microsoft Word one too. The Word file has grown by leaps and bounds through the years, because every time I came across something funny I would cut and paste it into this file. And I recently turned this file into a book. After all, I can't take this stuff with me when I "buy the farm" and wanted to share it with all you good people.

You should never have a day without laughter, and you also should never have a day when you don't make someone else laugh (or at least smile from ear to ear). Your sense of humor is one of your strongest assets, and it 's important to keep on using it. In my book, _Add Humor To Your Life; Add Life To Your Humor_, I have a 10 day program that will help you supercharge your humor. Okay, I'm a little bias – but I think this program is fantastic!

And, of course, one of the activities in this program is to establish your own "Silly File". But, with my new book, _The Funniest Book You Will Ever Read. Period!_, you have my _Silly File_ as a starter. What more could you want – thank you very much? If this all sounds like a shameless plug for my books, that's probably because it is. But I genuinely feel that these books will help you supercharge your humor and add zest to your life. Check them out at my Amazon Author page.

So, here are just a few snippets from my _silly file_:

The Dentist Visit

A man and his wife walked into a dentist's office. The man said to the dentist, "Doc, I'm in one heck of a hurry I have two buddies sitting out in my car waiting for us to go play golf, so forget about the anesthetic, I don't have time for the gums to get numb. I just want you to pull the tooth, and be done with it! We have a 10:00 AM tee time at the best golf course in town and it's 9:30 already... I don't have time to wait for the anesthetic to work!'

The dentist thought to himself, "My goodness, this is surely a very brave man asking to have his tooth pulled without using anything to kill the pain." So the dentist asks him, "Which tooth is it sir?"

The man turned to his wife and said, "Open your mouth Honey, and show him.

Tom's Inheritance

Tom was a single guy living at home with his father and working in the family business. When he found out he was going to inherit a fortune once his sickly father died, he decided he needed a wife with which to share his fortune.

One evening at an investment meeting, he spotted the most beautiful woman he had ever seen. Her natural beauty took his breath away.

"I may look like just an ordinary man," he said to her, "but in just a few years, my father will die, and I'll inherit 20 million dollars." Impressed, the woman obtained his business card.

Three days later, she became his stepmother. Women are so much better at estate planning than men.

The Story of Four Brothers

Four brothers left home for college, and they became successful doctors and lawyers. One evening, they chatted after having dinner together. They discussed the 95th birthday gifts they were able to give their elderly mother who moved to Florida.

The first said, "You know I had a big house built for Mama." The second said, "And I had a large theater built in the house."The third said, "And I had my Mercedes dealer deliver an SL600 to her."

The fourth said, "You know how Mama loved reading the Bible and you know she can't read anymore because she can't see very well. I met this preacher who told me about a cockatoo who could recite the entire Bible. It took ten preachers almost 8 years to teach him. I had to pledge to contribute $50,000 a year for five years to the church, but it was worth it . Mama only has to name the chapter and verse, and the parrot will recite it."

The other brothers were impressed. After the celebration Mama sent out her "Thank You" notes. She wrote: Milton , the house you built is so huge that I live in only one room, but I have to clean the whole house. Thanks anyway." "Marvin, I am too old to travel. I stay home; I have my groceries delivered, so I never use the Mercedes. The thought was good. Thanks." "Michael, you gave me an expensive theater with Dolby sound and it can hold 50 people, but all of my friends are dead, I've lost my hearing, and I'm nearly blind. I'll never use it. Thank you for the gesture just the same."

"Dearest Melvin, you were the only son to have the good sense to give a little thought to your gift. The chicken was delicious. Thank you so much."

Love, Mama

"Laughter is the shock absorber that eases the blows of life."

Early Signs of a Stroke

This may be the shortest page, but it also may be the most important. I've seen this a number of times and think it is so important for everyone to know. Too many people I have known have suffered strokes, but early detection and treatment these days can result in the prevention of permanent damage or death. Knowing the signs of a stroke may one day help you to save someone (maybe even yourself).

Commit these signs to memory. I hope you will never need them but, if the time ever comes, you'll be prepared.

If you suspect someone you are with is having a stroke:

- **Ask them to smile.**
- **Ask them to say a simple sentence and then repeat it.**
- **Ask them to raise their arms above their heads.**
- **Ask them to stick out their tongue. If it is crooked or leans either left or right, it is a clear indication of a stroke.**

If they cannot do any of these, call 911 right away. A quick response may save their life! Stay with them until help arrives.

One thing you may want to think about is to get some training in various first aid techniques. Every community has a number of options for this. Having a working knowledge of CPR, Heimlich Maneuvers, and other techniques may be a very valuable asset for you.

In our community (The Villages, Florida) there are a number of AED's (automated external defibrillators) and they have resulted in a number of lives saved. They allow a very quick response to heart attack victims from surrounding neighbors. If you think your community would benefit from these, contact your local Public Safety Department for details.

"You can't make everyone happy. You are not a jar of Nutella."

The Importance of Unlearning

Yes, I said "unlearning". Lifelong learning is one of the most powerful assets we have to stay young. But consider this quotation for a moment and let it sink in:

> **"To gain knowledge, learn something every day.**
> **To gain wisdom, unlearn something every day."**

Over the years, many of the things we learn and accept actually block us from bringing new ideas into our lives. When we attempt to expand our thinking, the paradigms that we have built about how things are "supposed to be" can severely limit our thinking. In my many years as a creative process consultant, I have seen some remarkable results from groups of people who were able to change the way they think. Quite often, these accepted rules are very simple. For example, it was long assumed that a car had one engine. Years ago, Audi engineers asked themselves "why?" – and the idea of hybrid vehicles was born. Just a simple unlearning and a whole new world of ideas opened up!

So what can you do about it? How can this help you "grow young"? What are some things you can "unlearn" today? Think of some of the assumptions and rules that now govern your life and see what happens if you can set these aside. Maybe you want to ask yourself, "What rule can I break today?"

Good luck and let me know if this worked for you.

And, speaking of learning, I just discovered something that may interest many of you. **United Health Care has something called the Learning Academy Courses** that looks pretty good. It's free, and you don't have to be one of their clients. I'm going to check some of these out – maybe you want to as well. Check it out at United Health Care.

"You can't steal second base if you never leave first base."

Happy Words

Our state of mind is often reflected in the words we use. If you tend to use "sad" words, it is likely that your demeanor will be sad. On the other hand, if you focus on using "happy" words, there's a good chance you will become a happy, humorous, and more attractive person. What kind of words do you tend to use? If your honest answer is not "happy words" then do your best to change this. Here are some happy words to get you started:

Affectionate	Ecstatic	Heavenly
Agreeable	Elated	Joy
Amazed	Enjoyable	Jubilant
Beautiful	Enthusiastic	Lively
Blessed	Excellent	Loved
Blissful	Excited	Lovely
Brilliant	Fabulous	Magnificent
Bubbly	Fantastic	Marvelous
Cheerful	Friendly	Optimistic
Comfortable	Glad	Perfect
Confident	Good	Pleased
Content	Grateful	Pleasure
Creative	Great	Satisfied
Delighted	Happiness	Spectacular
Delightful	Happy	Superb

Try to use as many of these as you can in the next few days and see what happens.

"The real happy person is the one who can enjoy the scenery on a detour".

My Observations on Life

A few years ago I published an article about my observations in the business world, and people loved it. If you'd like a copy of this let me know and I'll email it to you, because I'm such a nice guy. As I perused this article, it occurred to me that many of these observations apply to life in general, and may serve as learning experiences on how to change and grow young again. Let me share a few with you.

Observation #1

We tend to expend far more energy in solving problems than we do in creating new opportunities. We are a bit like ducks; great at paddling but a little shaky at flying. How might your life be different if you spent some time forgetting about problems and, instead, focusing on creating a great future?

Observation #2

Solutions to most problems often create more problems than they solve. Solving problems is like hanging wallpaper or pushing a cork into the water. If you've ever had the pleasure of hanging wallpaper you know it consists of getting the paper in the right position followed by chasing water bubbles around. When you push a bubble down it just comes up some place else. When you suppress a problem in your life, it just may emerge somewhere else. When you push a cork down into water it wants to push back. The harder you push it the harder it pushes back. The harder you push on problems, the more likely the push back may create problems of its own.

Observation #3

We tend to navigate through rear view mirrors. The strong relationship we tend to have with the past often limits our ability to create more interesting, and exciting futures. Try to put some duct tape over your rear view mirror and see if anything changes.

Observation #4

We spend much too much time and energy whining and moaning. People love to complain about the weather (which they can't change) and their personal and work lives (which they can change). What would happen if we could channel the energy we use to moan and whine towards some real change? In my past life as an expert in creative thinking I would often sponsor "whine and jeez parties" for my clients. This gave them the chance to get rid of all those pent up reasons to whine and, by the way, it was always a real blast to do this too. You may want to try this sometime. I'll even send you a list of things you can whine about.

Observation #5

Our viewpoints tend to be like those of a race horse with blinders. We see only what's right in front of us. There are huge possibilities outside this field of view that we miss seeing. How might your life change if you took off the blinders? Go ahead, take them off and take a good look at some things you've never noticed before.

Observation #6

For the most part, we love to stay in our comfort zones and not take too many chances. We are afraid to take chances because we are afraid we might fail. Failure and making mistakes tend to be frowned upon when, in fact, they are often the best road to success. The inventor of WD 40 gave his product that name because it was his 40th try at coming up with a perfect water displacement product (WD).

Observation #7

When we see the need for change we often just shake things up a bit and hope for the best. In organizations I use to refer to this as "the bird cage theory". We think of our situations as a cage full of birds sitting on their perches. . Every now and we give the cage a good shaking, and the birds fly around. When the shaking stops they all land on new perches, but everything else stays pretty much the same.

Observation #8

The things that got you to where you are today are usually not the things that will get you to the future. Few of us know how to "unlearn" some of the things that are getting in the way of future progress. Most of our energy is focused on "pushing today forward" and not "creating a great tomorrow". How might you really change your life if you could create a strong focus on the future?

Observation #9

There is a lot more talk than action. If things are not going well, it is difficult to change because we are busy trying to figure out why. When things are going well, it's sometimes even harder to effect change because the "If it ain't broke don't fix it" syndrome takes over.

I hope I haven't discouraged you with these observations. Try to put a positive spin on each of them and see if you can create a new, exciting future for yourself.

"There are secret opportunities hidden inside every failure."

~ 90 ~

What Goes Around Comes Around

I'd like to share a story with you that I just found in my archives. There's an old saying that "What goes around, comes around." This story is a perfect illustration of that, and lays the groundwork for something we all should try to do in our lives.

One day a man saw an old lady, stranded on the side of the road, but even in the dim light of day, he could see she needed help. So he pulled up in front of her Mercedes and got out. His Pontiac was still sputtering when he approached her.

Even with the smile on his face, she was worried. No one had stopped to help for the last hour or so. Was he going to hurt her? He didn't look safe; he looked poor and hungry. He could see that she was frightened, standing out there in the cold. He knew how she felt. It was those chills which only fear can put in you. He said, "I'm here to help you, ma'am. Why don't you wait in the car where it's warm? By the way, my name is Bryan Anderson."

Well, all she had was a flat tire, but for an old lady, that was bad enough. Bryan crawled under the car looking for a place to put the jack, skinning his knuckles a time or two. Soon he was able to change the tire. But he had to get dirty and his hands hurt.

As he was tightening up the lug nuts, she rolled down the window and began to talk to him. She told him that she was from St. Louis and was only just passing through. She couldn't thank him enough for coming to her aid.

Bryan just smiled as he closed her trunk. The lady asked how much she owed him. Any amount would have been all right with her. She already imagined all the awful things that could have happened had he not stopped. Bryan never thought twice about being paid. This was not a job to him. This was helping someone in need, and God knows there were plenty, who had given him a hand in the past. He had lived his whole life that way, and it never occurred to him to act any other way.

He told her that if she really wanted to pay him back, the next time she saw someone who needed help, she could give that person the assistance they needed, and Bryan added, "And think of me."

He waited until she started her car and drove off. It had been a cold and depressing day, but he felt good as he headed for home, disappearing into the twilight.

A few miles down the road the lady saw a small cafe. She went in to grab a bite to eat, and take the chill off before she made the last leg of her trip home. It was a dingy looking restaurant. Outside were two old gas pumps. The whole scene was unfamiliar to her. The waitress came over and brought a clean towel to wipe her wet hair. She had a sweet smile, one that even being on her feet for the whole day couldn't erase. The lady noticed the waitress was nearly eight months pregnant, but she never let the strain and aches change her attitude. The old lady wondered how someone who had so little could be so giving to a stranger. Then she remembered Bryan.

After the lady finished her meal, she paid with a hundred dollar bill. The waitress quickly went to get change for her hundred dollar bill, but the old lady had slipped right out the door. She was gone by the time the waitress came back. The waitress wondered where the lady could be. Then she noticed something written on the napkin.

There were tears in her eyes when she read what the lady wrote: "You don't owe me anything. I have been there too. Somebody once helped me out, the way I'm helping you. If you really want to pay me back, here is what you do, do not let this chain of love end with you." Under the napkin were four more $100 bills.

Well, there were tables to clear, sugar bowls to fill, and people to serve, but the waitress made it through another day. That night when she got home from work and climbed into bed, she was thinking about the money and what the lady had written. How could the lady have known how much she and her husband needed it? With the baby due next month, it was going to be hard... She knew how worried her husband was, and as he lay sleeping next to her, she gave him a soft kiss and whispered soft and low, "Everything's going to be all right. I love you, Bryan Anderson."

That's nice, isn't it? Keep this story in mind the next time you get a chance to help someone.

"Of All the paths you take in life, make sure a few of them are dirt."

Don't Mess With Seniors

A friend of mine sent me this little story of the $2.99 special and it occurred to me that it nicely illustrated how shrewd seniors can be. So I tossed in a few other illustrations that also prove that you should not mess with seniors. Enjoy!

The 2.99 Special.

We went to breakfast at a restaurant where the 'seniors' special' was two eggs, bacon, hash browns and toast for $2.99. 'Sounds good,' my wife said. 'But I don't want the eggs.' 'Then, I'll have to charge you $3.49 because you're ordering a la carte,' the waitress warned her. 'You mean I'd have to pay for not taking the eggs?' my wife asked incredulously. 'YES!' stated the waitress. 'I'll take the special then,' my wife said. 'How do you want your eggs?' the waitress asked. 'Raw and in the shell,' my wife replied. She took the two eggs home and baked a cake.

The Armed Robber

An armed hooded robber bursts into the Bank of Ireland and forces the tellers to load a sack full of cash. On his way out the door with the loot one brave Irish customer grabs the hood and pulls it off revealing the robber's face. The robber shoots the guy without hesitation!

He then looks around the bank to see if anyone else has seen him. One of the tellers is looking straight at him and the robber shoots him also. Everyone by now is very scared and looking down at the floor.

Did anyone else see my face?' calls the robber. There are a few moments of silence, then one elderly Irish gent, looking down, tentatively raises his hand and says:

'I think my wife may have caught a glimpse....'

Old Man from Idaho

An old man lived alone in Idaho. He wanted to spade his potato garden, but it was very hard work. His only son, Bubba, who used to help him, was in prison. The old man wrote a letter to his son and described his predicament.

Dear Bubba,
I am feeling pretty bad because it looks like I won't be able to plant my potato garden this year. I'm just getting too old to be digging up a garden plot. If you were here, all my

troubles would be over. I know you would dig the plot for me.
Love Dad

A few days later he received a letter from his son.

Dear Dad
For heaven's sake, dad, don't dig up that garden, that's where I Buried the
BODIES. Love Bubba

At AM the next morning, F.B.I. agents and local police showed up and dug up the entire area without finding any bodies. They apologized to the old man and left. That same day the old man received another letter from his son.

Dear Dad
Go ahead and plant the potatoes now. It's the best I could do under the
circumstances Love Bubba.

Elderly Man in Phoenix

An elderly man in Phoenix calls his son in New York and says, "I hate to ruin your day, but I have to tell you that your mother and I are divorcing, forty-five years of misery is enough."

"Pop, what are you talking about?" the son screams.

"We can't stand the sight of each other any longer, "the old man says. " We're sick of each other, and I'm sick of talking about this, so you call your sister in Chicago and tell her," and hangs up.

Frantic, the son calls his sister, who explodes on the phone. "Like heck they are getting divorced," she shouts, "I'll take care of this." She calls Phoenix immediately, and screams at the old man, "You are not getting divorced. Don't do a single thing until I get there. I'm calling my brother back, and we'll both be there tomorrow. Until then, don't do a thing, DO YOU HEAR ME?" and hangs up.

The old man hangs up the phone and turns to his wife. "Okay," he says. "They're coming for Thanksgiving and paying their own way"!

DON'T MESS WITH SENIORS!!! WE'VE been around the block more than once!

"If you change the way you look at things, the things you look at change."

Why You Should Sleep on Your Left Side

There are a number of very important reasons why we should always sleep on our left side. And a number of these are more important as we get older. It can have positive effects on our digestion, our backs, and even our hearts due to the positioning of the organs in our bodies.

I have always been amazed at the design of our bodies, but there is one thing that is lacking – an operating manual. If there were one, it would clearly state the proper sleeping position.

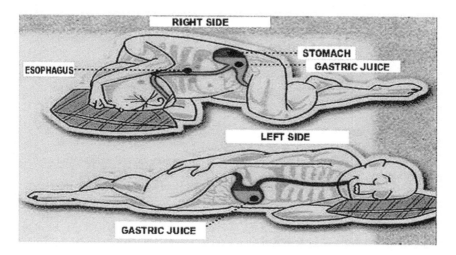

Here is a very simple look at the benefits I've found from various sources:

It prevents heartburn

Have you ever slept on your right side only to discover a good case of acid reflux, especially after a spicy or acidic meal? I certainly have. It's pretty clear in the above picture that sleeping on your left side results in gravity forcing your stomach acid into the pit of your stomach instead of sending it back up your esophagus, which occurs when you sleep on your right side.

It aids in digestion

Lying on your left side improves digestion by putting less strain on your liver. This, in turn, stimulates bile flow and increases nutrients absorption.

It clears lymph

The left side of the body is the dominant lymphatic side. The majority of the body's lymph fluid drains into the thoracic duct, located on the left side. Sleeping on your left side stimulates the drainage of toxins from the lymph nodes.

It can prevent snoring

Sleeping on your left side may also relieve sleep apnea and snoring. This position opens airways by keeping your tongue and throat muscles in a neutral position. In contrast, sleeping on your back pushes these muscles towards the back of your throat and causes distinct snoring noises as you struggle to breathe.

It may improve brain health

There is some research that suggests that sleeping on your left side helps your brain filter out waste which may even help prevent certain health conditions, like Alzheimer's.

It improves circulation

Sleeping on your left side improves blood circulation throughout the night. In fact, sleeping on your left side takes pressure off your vena cava (largest vein in the body), which is located on the right side of your body and supplies blood to the right side of your heart.

Which side do you sleep on? If you don't tend to sleep on your left side, it may be time to change this habit. If you have a hard time switching sides, simply place a body pillow on your right side to keep you from rolling over or keep a nightlight on the right side of your bed to naturally draw you towards the left.

Or you can also try keeping a pillow on your left side and placing it in between your knees and shoulders as if you were giving it a hug. That's even a better idea if that pillow is your sleeping partner.

Sleep tight!

"No one is remembered for being normal."

Renewing Your Friendships

One of my ongoing goals has been to make contact and renew relationships with as many old friends and relatives as I can. Sometimes I'm successful and sometimes not. Most of the time, it is very exciting reconnecting with old friends. And your friends are usually pretty excited to hear from you too. On occasion I find some are no longer living, which is a bummer. Either way, I highly recommend it.

So how do you go about doing this? Start by brainstorming a list of those you would like to contact. Begin with relatives (cousins, nieces, nephews, etc), and then with old friends. Think about childhood friends, high school and college buddies, service contacts, past neighbors, business associates, etc. If you have a large email address book like me, you may want to peruse this too. You may want to then prioritize this list.

Then allot a few minutes of your week to do some searching. Here are a few ways to start:

- Google their names. You may be surprised. While you are at it, Google your own name. I found out a lot about myself when I did that (most of it good).

- Search their names on social media (Facebook, LinkedIn, Google+, Twitter etc.).

- Go to the White Pages app and search. When you do this, knowing possible locations, ages, and some people who are connected to your friends will help you find them.

- If you have Email addresses, send them a note to see if they are still using this address. If they don't answer you it either means they are no longer at this address or maybe just don't want to hear from you.

Then it's just a matter of contacting your friends and reconnecting. Update their information, establish social media connections, put them in your address book (you may want to establish a special group for this), and stay in touch.

"Life is like riding a bicycle. To keep your balance you must keep moving."

Albert Einstein

Some Thoughts from Lou Holtz

A while back I had the pleasure of hearing Lou Holtz who spoke here in The Villages, Florida. If you ever get a chance to see him speak – take it! He was very entertaining, and has some very powerful and simple messages, especially for those of us in our mature years. He says **everything is either growing or dying**. And when we are at the top of our game, the tendency is to concentrate on maintaining, not growing. Interesting thought, isn't it? This has all sorts of implications for those of us interested in "growing young". Have you stopped thinking about growing? If so, see what you can do to change this.

Maintaining yourself is obviously not a bad thing. We need to pay attention to that, and there are a lot of good tips in this book to help you. But growing is a totally different animal. What are some of the things you can do to continue growing for the rest of your life?

His main message was that you need four things in your life:

- Something to do
- Someone to love
- Something to believe in, and
- Something to hope for

This message is so simple, and yet so powerful! How do you stand relative to these needs? Take a real serious look and see what changes you need to make.

He recalled when he developed a list of 108 things he wanted to do in his lifetime. He has completed 104 of these and he is in his 80's. I think he needs to add some to his list – you never want to complete that list. One of the things he said he wanted to do, but still hasn't, is "To run with the bulls – with a slower person". What a great line!

His three rules for growing are:

- Do what is right – avoid what is wrong.
- Do everything to the best of your ability.
- Show people you care.

Write this down and make it your motto today. Here are a couple of his quotations.

"We can win as soon as we run out of excuses for why we can't".

"It's good to be successful. But it's great to be significant".

Be Someone's Reason to Smile Today

There's an old song that goes something like this:

"Make someone happy, and you'll be happy too."

What a great piece of advice! In my books and presentations I often stress the importance of making others happy. When you make others happy, that happiness comes back to you in spades. Happiness is quite infectious – and it's an infection you want to pass on. And making others happy is not rocket science. It can be as easy as just smiling at people, and wishing them a nice day. It can be telling someone they have a nice smile, or a nice laugh. It can be sharing a funny line, joke, observation, or quotation that the situation brings to mind.

If you are somewhat of a natural outgoing person, you'll find this is pretty easy. If you are not (and I think many people fall into this category) you may find this more difficult. I suggest you work on it though. Next time you are out walking, shopping, or involved in any activity where you are among other people, go out of your way to smile at everyone you meet. Include a pleasant statement as well if you can. I assure you that you'll begin to really enjoy the experience. You will find that you will begin to enjoy brightening others lives – and you'll be surprised at how much you will brighten your own life.

If you know of someone who is unhappy, or having a difficult time, be their reason to smile, and the effect will be even more powerful. I saw a quotation recently that said:

"Be the Rainbow in Someone Else's Cloud."

What a powerful thought! Look for some opportunities to do this, and you will be rewarded.

Start each day by flashing a big smile at yourself in the mirror. This will give you the boost you need pass this on to others.

Keep on smiling!!

"Smile like a monkey with a new banana."

Remember our Veterans – A Wonderful Story

Being a Veteran, I am always on the lookout for things that show an appreciation for those who give so much for our country. This story is one that is well worth sharing. My hats off to teachers like this!

In September of 2005, on the first day of school, Martha Cothren, a history teacher at Robinson High School in Little Rock did something not to be forgotten. On the first day of school, with the permission of the school superintendent, the principal and the building supervisor, she removed all of the desks in her classroom. When the first period kids entered the room they discovered that there were no desks.

'Ms. Cothren, where are our desks?'

She replied, 'You can't have a desk until you tell me how you earn the right to sit at a desk.'

They thought, 'Well, maybe it's our grades.' 'No,' she said.

'Maybe it's our behavior.' She told them, 'No, it's not even your behavior.'

And so, they came and went, the first period, second period, third period. Still no desks in the classroom. Kids called their parents to tell them what was happening and by early afternoon television news crews had started gathering at the school to report about this crazy teacher who had taken all the desks out of her room.

The final period of the day came and as the puzzled students found seats on the floor of the desk-less classroom, Martha Cothren said, 'Throughout the day no one has been able to tell me just what he or she has done to earn the right to sit at the desks that are ordinarily found in this classroom. Now I am going to tell you.'

At this point, Martha Cothren went over to the door of her classroom and opened it. Twenty-seven (27) U.S. Veterans, all in uniform, walked into that classroom, each one carrying a school desk. The Vets began placing the school desks in rows, and then they would walk over and stand alongside the wall. By the time the last soldier had set the final desk in place those kids started to understand, perhaps for the first time in their lives, just how the right to sit at those desks had been earned

Martha said, 'You didn't earn the right to sit at these desks. These heroes did it for you. They placed the desks here for you. They went halfway around the world, giving up their education and interrupting their careers and families so you could have the freedom you have. Now, it's up to you to sit in them. It is your responsibility to learn, to be good students, to be good citizens. They paid the price so that you could have the freedom to get an education. Don't ever forget it.'

By the way, this is a true story. And this teacher was awarded the Veterans of Foreign Wars Teacher of the Year for the State of Arkansas in 2006. She is the daughter of a WWII POW.

Let us always remember the men and women of our military and the rights that they have won for us.

"America without its soldiers would be like God without his angels."

Quotations to Change Your Life

By now you should have gotten the hint that I love quotations. I include one in each post and I hope you enjoy them. Now let's take a look at some ways you can really put them to use.

- Pick one each day that you will use to guide you through the rough spots.
- Print and post one to your office wall – change often.
- Treat them like baseball cards and trade them with your friends.
- Stick a new one on the visor of your car everyday for the ride to work or recreation.
- Leave carefully chosen ones on the walls of your associates or boss to drop hints.
- Tape one under each chair before a meeting or gathering and have people read and discuss them.
- Use one in your email signature and change it often.
- Pass them out to strangers who look like they could use a real boost.
- Stick some on local bulletin boards.
- Use some as a screen saver on your computer.
- Put on your phone message.

So many quotations come with powerful messages that can have some very positive meaning to your life. Explore these possibilities by asking questions like:

- How might my life be different if I were to live by these words?

- How might I do to better if I lived by these words?

- What would change if I focused on carrying out the ideas in this quotation?

- How might I integrate the ideas in this quotation in a way that changes my behavior?

So here are a few of my current favorites to start you out. There are a lot of wonderful sources of quotes on the internet – just search around. I have become an avid user of Pinterest which allows you to create boards of things that interest you. And it might not surprise you that one of my boards contains my favorite quotes. Check them out at my Pinterest page, **pinterest.com/lindsaycollier**.

"Listen to the advice of older people. Not because they are right, but because they have the most experience being wrong."

"There are seven days in the week and someday isn't one of them."

"The harder you work, the luckier you get."

"Every flower must grow through dirt."

"You are not what you think you are but, what you think, you are."
Shirley Mclean

"He who wants milk should not stand in the middle of a pasture and wait for a cow to back up to him."

"The definition of insanity is when you keep doing the same thing over and over again, each time hoping for different results."

"Better to move forward and stumble than to stand still and grumble."

"You can't build a reputation on what you're going to do."

"What soap is to the body, laughter is to the soul."

"Whether you believe you can or believe you can't, you're absolutely right."

"I skate to where the puck is going to be, not to where it is."
Wayne Gretsky

Five Nutrients You Need

The older you get, the less efficient your body is at absorbing and using the nutrients you eat. Getting adequate nutrition is vital to overall health, function, quality of life and longevity.

Here are five nutrients that every older adult needs for better health — and how to make sure you're getting enough of each.

Protein

Older adults need to eat double the amount of protein that they needed in their younger years. They need to try and build each of their meals and snacks around a protein rich food. This means legumes (beans, lentils, and chickpeas) as well as dairy, eggs, fish, and lean meats. Using protein powder in your smoothies is another great source.

Calcium

Calcium is a bone-building all-star and is key during childhood (when your bones are growing) and older age (when bone mineral density and strength generally declines). You should gradually increase intake from 1,000 mg to 1,200 mg per day as you pass age 50. This is not because your body needs more, but because its ability to absorb and use calcium declines with age.

Unfortunately, many older adults experience stomach discomfort if they consume too much dairy and if that applies to you, opt for lactose-free milks.

Vitamin D

Vitamin D deficiency is incredibly common in people of all ages, but it tends to become even more severe at 65+ and is associated with a significantly greater risk of falling and suffering injuries from falls. Vitamin D is essential to both bone and muscle health and also linked to a reduced risk of age-related conditions including heart disease, cancer, and type 2 diabetes.

Next time you have a blood test ask to have your vitamin D levels checked. Once you know your levels, work with your physician to come up with a plan to meet your needs which may include dietary changes — eating more fatty fish, dairy, and eggs — or taking a supplement.

Fiber

Fiber needs actually increase as you get older and higher fiber intake is related to lower risk of heart disease.

Swap white bread and pasta for whole grain varieties, and make sure your diet is rich in legumes, fruits, and vegetables. You can also take a supplement like Metamucil or Citrucel to meet your daily requirements.

Water

Adequate water it's one of the most important things for your health. While the amount of water you need doesn't increase as you age, your body's thirst mechanism can get lazy. So it's important to drink water even if you aren't thirsty.

Keep a refillable water bottle with you whenever possible. Remember that fluid-filled foods (such as fruit and soup) as well as beverages (including tea and even coffee) hydrate you too.

The eight-glass-a-day rule is more of a suggestion these days. Fact is, your hydration needs vary depending on the foods you're eating, how much you're exercising, and any health conditions you may have. The one gauge that's pretty reliable: If your urine isn't clear, your body needs more water.

"When you were born, you were crying and everyone around you was smiling. Live your life to the fullest so that when you die, you're smiling and everyone around you is crying".

A Nice Story about Marbles

I got this from a friend and thought it would be nice to pass it on. It's a wonderful story with a lot of meaning.

I was at the corner grocery store buying some early potatoes. I noticed a small boy, delicate of bone and feature, ragged but clean, hungrily appraising a basket of freshly picked green peas. I paid for my potatoes but was also drawn to the display of fresh green peas. I am a pushover for creamed peas and new potatoes.

Pondering the peas, I couldn't help overhearing the conversation between Mr. Miller (the store owner) and the ragged boy next to me. 'Hello Barry, how are you today'? 'H'lo, Mr. Miller. Fine, thank ya. Jus' admirin' them peas. They sure look good'. 'They are good, Barry. How's your Ma'? 'Fine. Gittin' stronger alla' time'.

'Good. Anything I can help you with?' 'No, Sir. Jus' admirin' them peas'. 'Would you like to take some home?' asked Mr. Miller. 'No, Sir. Got nuthin' to pay for 'em with'.

'Well, what have you to trade me for some of those peas?' 'All I got's my prize marble here'. 'Is that right? Let me see it', said Miller. 'Here 'tis. She's a dandy'. 'I can see that. Hmm mmm, only thing is this one is blue and I sort of go for red. Do you have a red one like this at home?' the store owner asked. 'Not zackley but almost'.

'Tell you what. Take this sack of peas home with you and next trip this way let me look at that red marble'. Mr. Miller told the boy. 'Sure will. Thanks Mr. Miller'.

Mrs. Miller, who had been standing nearby, came over to help me. With a smile she said, 'There are two other boys like him in our community, all three are in very poor circumstances. Jim just loves to bargain with them for peas, apples, tomatoes, or whatever.

When they come back with their red marbles, and they always do, he decides he doesn't like red after all and he sends them home with a bag of produce for a green marble or an orange one, when they come on their next trip to the store'.

I left the store smiling to myself, impressed with this man. A short time later I moved to Colorado, but I never forgot the story of this man, the boys, and their bartering for marbles.

Several years went by, each more rapid than the previous one. Just recently I had occasion to visit some old friends in that Idaho community and while I was there learned that Mr. Miller had died. They were having his visitation that evening and knowing my friends wanted to go, I agreed to accompany them. Upon arrival at the mortuary we fell into line to meet the relatives of the deceased and to offer whatever words of comfort we could.

Ahead of us in line were three young men. One was in an army uniform and the other two wore nice haircuts, dark suits and white shirts...all very professional looking. They approached Mrs. Miller, standing composed and smiling by her husband's casket.

Each of the young men hugged her, kissed her on the cheek, spoke briefly with her and moved on to the casket. Her misty light blue eyes followed them as, one by one; each young man stopped briefly and placed his own warm hand over the cold pale hand in the casket. Each left the mortuary awkwardly, wiping his eyes.

Our turn came to meet Mrs. Miller. I told her who I was and reminded her of the story from those many years ago and what she had told me about her husband's bartering for marbles. With her eyes glistening, she took my hand and led me to the casket. 'Those three young men who just left were the boys I told you about'. They just told me how they appreciated the things Jim 'traded' them. Now, at last, when Jim could not change his mind about color or size....they came to pay their debt'.

'We've never had a great deal of the wealth of this world,' she confided, 'but right now, Jim would consider himself the richest man in Idaho'. With loving gentleness she lifted the lifeless fingers of her deceased husband. Resting underneath were three exquisitely shined red marbles.

The Moral

We will not be remembered by our words, but by our kind deeds. Life is not measured by the breaths we take, but by the moments that take our breath away.

"It's not what you gather in life but what you scatter in life that tells you what kind of life you have lived."

Focus On Cholesterol

Quite early in my life (probably my late thirties), a cholesterol screening showed that I had an impending problem. That later developed into a problem with heart disease (I'll spare the details here). It was pretty much heredity caused since I had a very healthy lifestyle. I remember my doctor telling me that I could have eaten only rice all my life, and would still have a problem.

It's so important for seniors to have periodic blood tests and, if you have a good health care plan and a good doctor, this will happen. There are a lot of indicators on these tests, but perhaps the most important are your cholesterol readings. However, these can get a bit confusing.

Results of your blood test will come in the forms of numbers. Here is how to interpret your cholesterol numbers. The first thing you need to know is that the numbers by themselves are not enough to predict your risk of heart problems or to determine what you need to do to lower that risk. They are, instead, one part of a larger equation that includes your age, your blood pressure, your smoking status, and your use of blood pressure medicines. Your doctor will use this information to calculate your 10-year risk for serious heart problems. Then the two of you will develop a strategy for reducing that risk.

Screening and control of the following indicators should be a high priority with you if you tend towards having high cholesterol.

LDL Cholesterol

LDL cholesterol can build up on the walls of your arteries and increase your chances of getting heart disease. That is why LDL cholesterol is referred to as 'bad' cholesterol. The lower your LDL cholesterol number, the lower your risk.

For most people an LDL below 100 is considered healthy. If your LDL is 190 or more, it is considered very high. Your doctor will most likely recommend a statin in addition to making healthy lifestyle choices. Statins are medicines that can help lower cholesterol levels.

You may also need to take a statin even though your LDL level is lower than 190. After figuring your 10-year risk, your doctor will recommend a percentage by which you should try to lower your LDL level through diet, exercise, and medication if necessary.

HDL Cholesterol

HDL cholesterol is referred to as 'good' cholesterol and a higher number means lower risk. This is because HDL cholesterol protects against heart disease by taking the 'bad' cholesterol out of your blood and keeping it from building up in your arteries. A statin can slightly increase your HDL but exercise is a major contributor to it. **You should aim for a reading over 60 for this indicator.**

Triglycerides

Triglycerides are the form in which most fat exists in food and the body. The body converts excess calories, sugar, and alcohol into triglycerides, a type of fat that is carried in the blood and stored in fat cells throughout the body. People who are overweight, inactive, smokers, or heavy drinkers tend to have high triglycerides, as do those who eat a very high-carb diet A high triglyceride level has been linked to higher risk of coronary artery disease. **The goal is to keep this indicator less than 150.** A triglycerides score of 150 or higher puts you at risk for metabolic syndrome, which is linked to heart disease and diabetes

Total Cholesterol

Your total blood cholesterol is a measure of LDL cholesterol, HDL cholesterol, and other lipid components. Your doctor will use your total cholesterol number when determining your risk for heart disease and how best to manage it.

Several factors can make you more likely to develop high cholesterol.

- A diet high in saturated fats and cholesterol
- A family history of high cholesterol
- Being overweight or obese
- Aging

If you have a tendency toward unhealthy levels of cholesterol you should work with your doctor to develop a plan to eat healthier, exercise more, and get on the medicines that will bring your indicators to healthy levels.

"Live your life and forget your age."

Texting for Seniors - A Comical Look at Growing Old

Aging is something that is going to happen whether you like it or not. So why not take a comical look at it? I live in what may be called a retirement community where there are a lot of 'snowbirds'. But the number of folks who live there year-round is increasing, and they often refer to themselves as FROGS. What that means is that they are 'here till they croak'. They also sometimes refer to the community as 'God's Waiting Room'.

A while back, I bought myself a tee shirt at a gift shop in Tarpon Springs, Florida (a wonderful place to visit by the way). This shirt was called "Texting for Seniors" and I just feel compelled to share it with you. So, here is some of the texting shorthand for seniors:

CUATSC – See You at the Senior Center

DWI – Driving While Incontinent

WWNO – Walker Wheels Need Oil

IMHO – Is My hearing Aid On?

LOL – Living on Lipitor

ROFL –CGU – Rolling on the Floor Laughing – Can't Get Up

GGLKI – Gotta Go, Laxative Kicking In

ATD – At the Doctor's

BYOT – Bring Your Own Teeth

FWIW – Forgot Where I Was.

GGPBL – Gotta Go, Pacemaker Battery Low

LMDO – Laughing My Dentures Out

TOT – Texting on Toilet

BFF – Best Friends Funeral

Okay, I have a little space left here, so here are a couple of senior jokes:

Morris, an 82 year-old man, went to the doctor to get a physical. A few days later, the doctor saw Morris walking down the street with a gorgeous young woman on his arm.

A couple of days later, the doctor spoke to Morris and said, 'You're really doing great, aren't you?' Morris replied, 'Just doing what you said, Doc: 'Get a hot mamma and be cheerful.'

The doctor said, 'I didn't say that. I said, 'You've got a heart murmur; be careful.'

An aging man had serious hearing problems for a number of years. He went to the doctor and the doctor was able to have him fitted for a set of hearing aids that allowed the gentleman to hear 100%. The elderly gentleman went back in a month to the doctor and the doctor said, 'Your hearing is perfect. Your family must be really pleased that you can hear again.'

The gentleman replied, 'Oh, I haven't told my family yet.
I just sit around and listen to the conversations. I've changed my will three times!'

Hospital regulations require a wheel chair for patients being discharged. However, while working as a student nurse, I found one elderly gentleman already dressed and sitting on the bed with a suitcase at his feet, who insisted he didn't need my help to leave the hospital.

After a chat about rules being rules, he reluctantly let me wheel him to the elevator. On the way down I asked him if his wife was meeting him. 'I don't know,' he said. 'She's still upstairs in the bathroom changing out of her hospital gown.'

Hope this brought a smile to your day!

"Old age is always 15 years older than I am."

Shedding Pounds for Seniors

In my younger days it seemed very easy to lose weight. If I found I was getting a bit on the hefty side, I would just exercise a little more and eat a little less and those abs of steel would come back into view. As we get older this becomes much more difficult. I usually tell people that I still have my abs of steel, but I just like to protect them with a couple of extra layers.

For us mature folks, weight is easy to gain, and sometimes hard to lose. Shedding pounds does not necessarily require a complete diet and exercise overhaul. Just changing a few of your habits might be the answer. Here are a few habits you might want to adopt that take a minimal amount of effort.

Stay on the move as much as you can. You may want to invest in an activity tracker which will help you to set some goals and see how you are doing. Walking is one of the best things for you, so always include time in your day for this. Have a formal workout program if you can as well. Include some cardio and strength exercises, but don't overdo it. You're not trying to win a body beautiful contest, you're just trying to stay fit.

Eat water rich foods. Eating foods that contain a good amount of water, such as fruits, vegetables, or broth based soups can fill you up. This will leave you less likely to overeat on more calorie-dense foods. Try starting your meal with a broth based soup or add two or three leaves of lettuce and more tomato on your sandwich. And, of course, drink more water.

Eat protein rich foods, especially in the morning. Eating a protein-rich meal in the morning can set you up for a whole day of healthy eating. You may also want to have some protein powder available to supplement some of your meals (especially smoothies).

If you find yourself gaining weight DO NOT buy bigger clothes or begin wearing stretchable sweat pants. Doing this is just a form of accepting your weight gain. Instead of this set your goal to bring yourself back to the point where your clothes will fit you. Your goal is not to lose weight; it is to get your clothes back. Think of all the money you will save not having to buy new clothes.

Try to change your eating habits and rearrange your fridge and food cabinets so that the healthy foods are the ones easiest to get to. Reduce the amount of unhealthy snack foods in your diet and place them in areas that are more difficult to access. Make it a habit to check the ingredients of the snack foods you buy and shy away from those that look unhealthy (and that's probably most of them).

Be aware of your food portions. Many of us have a tendency to serve up portions of food that are well beyond what we need. If you are snacking from a large bag of chips you will likely eat a lot more than you should. It may be better to purchase the small portion bags which will give you a built-in control. And, when your plates are too full, you don't have to finish everything – despite what you mother told you. When I feel full I usually save the rest for tomorrow's lunch. I also find it useful to buy the cheaper family sized packages of meats and other foods and portion out smaller sized servings in individual baggies.

You may want to try and set your weight goals based on lab readings. Instead of telling yourself you want to lose a certain amount of pounds, tell yourself you want to lower your blood pressure or reduce your cholesterol readings. When you start eating a little better for the health issue, before you know it, a couple of pounds may be coming off. And the incentive to get these lab readings correct might be much stronger than that of just taking off pounds.

Finally, take advantage of programs offered by your health plan. If your plan offers free **Silver Sneakers** you're crazy if you don't take advantage of it. Here's what you get:

- Free gym membership at more than 14,000 gyms and fitness centers across the nation
- Free gym fitness classes led by certified instructors who specialize in working with older adults
- Free community fitness classes that range from tai chi to boot camp to yoga
- Unlimited access to any participating location or class in the Silver Sneakers network

Many plans offer free consultation with a nutritionist and you should also take advantage of this.

Here's to your health!

"When you change the way you look at things, the things you look at change."
Wayne Dyer

Your Life as an Iceberg

I have long thought that icebergs were great metaphors for life. I used them extensively in my consulting as an expert in creativity and innovation. What makes icebergs such an intriguing metaphor is the fact that such a small part of them appears above the surface. The so-called tip of the iceberg is what we see, but most of its mass is below the surface. This metaphor has all sorts of implications for you as you look more closely at your own life experience.

We tend to deal with those things above the surface that we can see. The part that *lies beneath the surface* tends to be ignored, but it doesn't go away – it comes back to get us eventually. People that have tried to deal with change have often been blocked in their attempts because they failed to change some of the powerful underlying assumptions and behaviors that influenced their results. If you shear off the tip of the iceberg, does the bottom go away?

- How might you define the part of you that exists above the surface?
- What are some of the things in your life that exist below the surface?
- What is the impact of some of those things below the surface on your life?
- What actions might be necessary to deal with these issues?

In dealing with your life challenges, there is a lot that lies beneath the surface. If we don't work on that it will likely sink us. Think of your task as being to melt the iceberg (or at least partially melt it). You need to melt equal proportions of the tip and the mass below – otherwise it will become very unstable. For every issue that you deal with that is above the surface, you need to deal with a multiple proportions of what's below.

Draw a picture of an iceberg and jot down some of the things in your life that are within its tip. Then identify as many things as you can that exist below the surface. What does this tell you about the stability (or instability) of your current situation? Most importantly, what possible changes does this suggest?

Try several iterations of this exercise and see what ideas come to mind as to things you might do to make your next 50 years your best 50 years.

And watch out for approaching ships!

"Inhale the future, exhale the past."

Live Your Life the Same Way Your Heart Gives You Life

It never ceases to amazing that our bodies are incredible engineering marvels! Take the heart as an example. The heart, lungs, arteries, and veins work constantly to provide life to the body. Oxygenated blood is pumped by the heart through the arteries to the entire body and provides nourishment to cells. It is returned to the lungs to pick up more oxygen and then back to the heart to start the cycle over again. It does this by beating 86,400 times per day! This is referred to as the cardio-thoracic system.

Years ago I found that there were some issues with my heart and it resulted in some pretty serious heart by-pass surgery. While recovering, I spent a lot of time thinking about how the cardio-thoracic system is a great metaphor for life. The question in my mind was, how does this system of our hearts, arteries, lungs, blood, and cells emulate the way we should lead our lives. Like I've said before, I like to turn negative experiences into learning experiences.

In the cardio-thoracic system a common problem is the build-up of blockages in the arteries typically caused by cholesterol. The arteries transferring blood become narrowed with cholesterol deposits and may even become totally blocked. Sometimes small detour arteries are created around the obstruction. In my case I was physically very active and tests showed that I had some pretty nice detours around the blockages. But sooner or later these blockages manifest themselves as pain when the system can't get the blood flow it needs. In times of high physical or mental stress the body calls for more oxygenated blood and the system can't respond. The result might be pain, an attack, or a stroke.

With all this in mind here are a couple of questions to ask yourself based on this system as a metaphor:

> What are some things that are blockages in your current thinking about your future?

> What are some of the detours you have managed to build around these blockages?

The main choices you have when there is significant enough blockage within the arteries to cause concern are:

Living with the pain. This pain is commonly referred to as *angina* and more than a few people live with this pain. This seems like a good short-term option but, unless there is a reversal of whatever is causing the pain in the first place, things will ultimately get worse. The objective here is to stay comfortable by not taking any risks.

> Is there pain in your life that you have decided to just live with?

Displace or Remove the blockage. A common method, *angio-plasti*, is to push aside the blockage in the arteries. This is suitable only in cases where the blockage is not too severe. A balloon is inflated within the artery at the blockage site and the plaque is pushed against the artery wall with a stent put in place to hold it there. What is a life equivalent to this? I think we often displace or temporarily remove things in our lives that are holding us back in hopes that they will never return. Guess what? They return! Sooner or later the blockage will again develop at the same site and probably at other sites as well.

Are there some things in your life that you have just temporarily pushed aside?

Create new roads around the blockage. In this case, new arteries (borrowed from other parts of the body) are used to by-pass areas of extreme blockage. It's pretty invasive but provides a fairly long-term fix if the cause of the blockage is removed. Are the blockages severe enough to warrant something this invasive?

Are there some things in your life that warrant some brand new detours?

Reverse what is causing the problem in the first place. All the options so far suffer from a similar, and critical, problem. If nothing is done to reverse what caused the problem in the first place it will very likely return. Each successive method just gives you a little more time. For the long term there may be a need for a total lifestyle change.

What changes can you make in your life that will permanently keep you from any blockages to attaining your dreams?

Wow – that was pretty deep. Let's look at something a lot lighter.

"There is nothing more beautiful than the way the ocean keeps kissing the shore line no matter how many times it's turned away."

The Ape Story

Here's a story I used often while helping organization create breakthrough in thinking about their future. It may have some interesting implications on how you think of your own future.

In a cage there are five apes. In the cage hangs a banana on a string over some stairs. Before long, one ape will go to the stairs and start to climb towards the banana, but as soon as he touches the stairs, all the apes are sprayed with cold water.

After a while, another ape makes an attempt with the same result and all the apes are sprayed with water. After another while, if an ape tries to climb the stairs, the other apes will act to prevent it.

Now, remove one ape from the cage and replace it with a new one. The new ape sees the banana and wants to climb the stairs. To his horror, all the other apes attack him. After another attempt and another attack, he knows that if he tries to climb the stairs, he will be assaulted.

Next, remove another of the original five apes and replace it with a new one. The newcomer goes to the stairs and is attacked. The previous newcomer takes part in the punishment with enthusiasm.

Replace another ape with a new one. The new one makes it to the stairs and is attacked as well. Two of the four apes that beat him have no idea why they were not permitted to climb the stairs, or why they are participating in the beating of the newest ape.

After replacing the fourth and fifth original apes, all the apes that have been sprayed with cold water have been replaced. Nevertheless, no ape ever again approaches the stairs.

Why not? Because they all think that's the way it's always been done around here, and none of them question it.

Are there some things in your life that you do because you think, that's the way it's always been done? I bet you can find a few of these and, when you do, ask yourself how you can change it.

"Forever is composed of 'Nows'."
Emily Dickenson

How Your Body Talks to You. Some Pains You Shouldn't Ignore

The older we get, the more we experience physical pain. That's pretty normal and not always a bad thing. Your body might just be telling you to slow down and take it easy. Pain that you feel after exerting yourself that goes away after a while should not be of too much concern. However, there are some pains that should not be ignored. Obviously, a crushing chest pain, a terrible headache, or a sharp intensifying stomach pain is something to be dealt with immediately. Here are a few less obvious pains you should ignore

Persistent neck pain. We all have neck pain from time to time and usually it is easily cured by a warm compress. But if it doesn't resolve itself within a few weeks it should be checked out. It could be signaling a greater problem.

Wrist pain that extend to the hands. Some wrist pain is a result of Osteoarthritis which may not be too severe, but will worsen with age. Rheumatoid arthritis is more severe and it tends to start in the hands and wrists before moving to other joints in the body.

Back pain accompanied by other symptoms. Back pain is very common among seniors and the general rule is that, if it goes away on its own within 6 weeks, you need not worry. If accompanied by other symptoms such as fever, night sweats, weight loss, bladder or bowel incontinence, it may signal a bigger problem and you should seek advice.

Knee pain when you walk. If the pain is persistent, you should see your doctor. It could be osteoarthritis, bursitis, or just a problem like flat feet putting extra stress on your knee.

Hip pain when your leg is lifted. For seniors, hips seem to create the most problems. You can fracture a hip without even knowing it just by landing hard on a leg. Hip fractures have also been known to cause blood clots that can flake off and travel to the lungs which could be fatal if not caught in time. You definitely need to see your doctor on this one.

Sudden Pain in Your Big Toe. If there is nothing you see that might cause pain in your toe (bunions, hammertoes etc.) then there is a good chance of gout. This is a build-up of uric acid crystals in the blood which can cause very severe pain. It seems to favor big toes, but it can also settle in your knee. I speak from experience here. The good news is that it can be treated with generic medicine.

"Anyone who keeps the ability to see beauty never grows old."
Franz Kafka

Feeding Your Brain

A major part of staying young involves keeping your brain active and healthy. Giving your brain daily workouts is every bit as important as working the body. Find ways that are fun for working the brain.

As far as mental workouts are concerned, there are lots of choices, especially if you have a smart phone, IPad, or similar device. Cross word puzzles, jigsaw puzzles, Sudoku, Words with Friends, and other brain booster apps are readily available. Mix it up between word challenges (like crosswords), logic (like Sudoku), and visual (like puzzles).

Have you noticed that the *brain booster* book sections in the most bookstores are getting bigger? Go to that section of your favorite bookstore and pick up a few of these books. There are also a number of brain booster apps and games for your IPad, smart phone or other similar device. Most of these are free but in some cases you may have to fork over a whole $.99 to get an add-free version. Choose games and puzzles that really challenge you, and stretch your thinking like a rubber band – not just the ones you can easily solve. As a matter of fact, the best ones might be those that you can't quite solve. When that is the case you know you are taking yourself right to the edge. And the more you take yourself to the edge, the higher your chances are to eventually extend beyond that edge. And, like a rubber band, the more it is stretched, the more pliable it becomes.

Most newspaper puzzles start on Monday with the easiest and get more difficult as the week goes on. Challenge yourself to get through the whole week with a particular puzzle. Give me a call if you get to the point of solving Saturday's puzzle and let me know what your secret is. I've never been able to come even close to solving Saturday's crossword, but maybe someday. I'll keep on trying. Also, challenge yourself to learn some brand new skills that will help you stretch your thinking while adding a little zest to your life.

A part of your mental work out should also be to read as often as you can. You may be able to find some learning possibilities on the TV, but sometimes it's just best to turn it off and open a good book or magazine. If you are a compulsive TV watcher make sure you spend some time on the learning channels. The Jerry Springer show is not one of them. Keep a variety in your reading lists to include fiction, non-fiction, short stories, auto-biographies, history, magazines etc. And you may want to try your hand at writing too. Most people don't look at themselves as being authors but you may surprise yourself. Once you begin writing it seems to open up the floodgates of your mind and it becomes quite addictive. And you just may find that you are smarter than you thought you were – as I did.

"A strong person smiles in trouble, gathers strength from distress, and grows brave by reflection."

It's Nappy Time

Have you found that you and your friends have been saying, "It's my nappy time" more frequently lately? I have to be honest, the older I get, the more I need a nap from time to time. But, as I think back to my younger days, I have always been prone to napping – except then I called it a "power snooze". Does this sound familiar? Actually napping is very good for you, no matter what your age. I remember in my working days that there were a few folks that spent their lunch time snoozing. And they seemed to be the same ones that were more energized all afternoon.

It turns out that napping can actually serve as a self-improvement tool. It can increase not only our health but our intelligence and productivity as well. Famous leaders like Edison, Churchill, JFK, and Napoleon were ardent nappers, and they did okay.

So why is napping so good for you?

It keeps you alert. When you are the point of almost dozing off a nap is the best thing for you. This is especially important if you are engaging in an activity such as driving where falling asleep could have grave consequences. They say that a 40 minute nap can increase alertness by 100%, but sometimes 20 minutes will even suffice. I find that whenever I have an event coming up, a quick nap just before attending makes a big difference.

It has a great effect on learning and memory. I write and do a lot of presentations and have found that taking a short nap just prior to these tasks is very beneficial. When you are worn down your working memory and learning capabilities are at their minimum, and a short nap can make a world of difference. Remember when you or your children were in Kindergarten and napping was a part of their day? There was a reason for that other than just getting the kids out of the teacher's hair for a while.

It can improve your overall health. Napping gives your brain a chance to rest and your body a chance to heal. When you sleep or nap you release a growth hormone which boosts your immune system, reduces stress and anxiety, and aids in muscle repair and weight loss. They say it also primes your sexual function as well. That alone seems to be a good enough reason for me to nap.

It reduces stress and improves our mood. If you have ever had children you will remember that, whenever a child was misbehaving the excuse was usually, "He's just overtired." Our moods can change quite drastically due to lack of sleep, and a short nap can change that. Napping is also a great anti-stress tool.

It stimulates your senses and your creativity. After napping you often realize that your senses are much sharper. Things may taste better, colors may be more vivid, and ideas may be clearer. After waking from a sound sleep these things are pretty obvious. But a short nap may also give your senses and creativity a real boost.

So, now that you know how valuable napping can be for you, what's keeping you from engaging in some "nappy time"? When is the best time to nap? I think any time you feel the need is the best time, but perhaps your lifestyle dictates that it's best to just find a time that fits your schedule and make it a daily experience.

If you have trouble napping find yourself a very dull book, sit back, relax, and start reading. You'll be asleep in minutes. Rocking chairs usually work too. I personally find it very relaxing and soothing to put the earphones on with some gentle jazz or classical music. And here is some advice I recently saw on a sign outside a church:

Having Trouble Sleeping? Try One of Our Sermons.

Enjoy your snooze!

"Your mind is a garden. Your thoughts are seeds.
You can grow flowers or you can grow weeds."

Some Words of Wisdom

The following was sent to me by a friend, and it's just too good not to pass on. There's some great 'straight from the heart' advice here and, unfortunately, I have no idea where it came from.

As I've aged, I've become kinder to myself, and less critical of myself. I've become my own friend.

I have seen too many dear friends leave this world too soon; before they understood the great freedom that comes with aging.

Whose business is it if I choose to read, or play, on the computer, until 4 AM, or sleep until noon? I will dance with myself to those wonderful tunes of the 50, 60 & 70's, and if I, at the same time, wish to weep over a lost love, I will.

I will walk the beach in a swim suit that is stretched over a bulging body, and will dive into the waves, with abandon, if I choose to, despite the pitying glances from the jet set. They, too, will get old.

I know I am sometimes forgetful. But there again, some of life is just as well forgotten. And, I eventually remember the important things.

Sure, over the years, my heart has been broken. How can your heart not break when you lose a loved one, or when a child suffers, or even when somebody's beloved pet gets hit by a car?

But, broken hearts are what give us strength, and understanding, and compassion. A heart never broken is pristine and sterile, and will never know the joy of being imperfect.

I am so blessed to have lived long enough to have my hair turning gray, and to have my youthful laughs be forever etched into deep grooves on my face. So many have never laughed, and so many have died before their hair could turn silver.

As you get older, it is easier to be positive. You care less about what other people think. I don't question myself anymore. I've even earned the right to be wrong.

So, to answer your question, I like being old. It has set me free. I like the person I have become. I am not going to live forever, but while I am still here, I will not waste time lamenting what could have been, or worrying about what will be. And I shall eat dessert every single day (if I feel like it).

"I get enough exercise just by pushing my luck."

Some Smile Quotations

Here a few of the "smile quotations" from my book, **Add Humor To Your Life; Add Life To Your Humor**. See how each of these might help you access your sense of humor. Add some to your email signature, put some on your car visor, paste one on your refrigerator, hang one from your nose – whatever suits you. In the morning, think about how this quote could make your day. You may find some duplicate quotes in this book but don't worry, seeing them twice won't hurt you.

After every storm the sun will smile; for every problem there is a solution, and the soul's indefeasible duty is to be of good cheer. – William R. Alger

You're never fully dressed without a smile. – Martin Charnin

A smile is happiness you'll find right under your nose. – Tom Wilson

"I was smiling yesterday, I am smiling today, and I will smile tomorrow, simply because life is too short to cry for anything." – Santosh Kalwar

Remember even though the outside world might be raining, if you keep on smiling, the sun will soon show its face and smile back at you. – Anna Lee

"Sometimes your joy is the source of your smile, but sometimes your smile can be the source of your joy." – Thich Nhat Hanh

When I look out at the people, and they look at me, and they're smiling, then I know that I'm loved. That is the time when I have no worries, no problems. – Etta James

A well-developed sense of humor is the pole that adds balance to your steps as you walk the tightrope of life. – William Arthur Ward

If I had no sense of humor, I would long ago have committed suicide. – Gandhi

The world always looks brighter from behind a smile.

Always remember to be happy because you never know who's falling in love with your smile.

"If I can see pain in your eyes, then share with me your tears. If I can see joy in your eyes, then share with me your smile." – Santosh Kalwar

Use your smile to change the world; don't let the world change your smile.

Never regret something that once made you smile.

You are somebody's reason to smile.

The more I live, the more I think that humor is the saving sense. – Jacob August

Riis Humor is mankind's greatest blessing. – Mark Twain

Every smile makes you a day younger. – Chinese Proverb

Seven days without laughter make one weak.

The secret source of humor itself is not joy, but sorrow. – Mark

Twain Do not take life seriously. You'll never get out of it alive.

People do not quit playing because they get old. They get old because they quite playing.

Laughter is like changing a baby's diaper. It doesn't change things permanently but it makes it better for a while.

It's never too late to have a happy childhood. You are only young once, but you can be immature all your life

Laughter is the shock absorber that eases the blows of life.

Those who bring sunshine into the lives of others cannot keep it from themselves.

Some people grin and bear it. Others smile and change it.

Laughter is the shortest distance between two people. – Victor Borge

There is no cosmetic for beauty like happiness. – Lady Blessington

With the fearful strain that is on me night and day, if I did not laugh, I should die. – Abraham Lincoln

A day without laughter is a day wasted.- Charlie Chaplin

More of the Funniest People I've Ever Known

In my book, **Add Humor To Your Life; Add Life To Your Humor**, one of the Appendices is a summary of all the funniest people I've ever known along with links to some of their funniest routines. I've had some folks tell me that this Appendix alone is worth the price of the book. And, I must say, it's a blast! One of the things I suggest in my book is to take time out every now and then for "humor breaks". Well, here's your opportunity for some humor breaks which should leave you smiling ear to ear.

Here are four more of the funniest people I've ever known:

Don Rickles

Normally I wouldn't put a comedian on this list who's major punch line is alienating people. He was a master at this, and did it in such a way that made everyone laugh – even if they were the butt of his jokes. Start by looking up these two on YouTube:

Don Rickles Roasts Ronald Regan

Don Rickles Roasts Sammy Davis Jr.

Rodney Dangerfield

Rodney was the master at self-effacing comedy. His line, "I get no respect" will go down in history. Here are a couple of his YouTube videos, and a few of his best quips:

Rodney Dangerfield Live

Rodney Dangerfield Stand Up

My wife only has sex with me for a purpose. Last night she used me to time an egg.

Last night my wife met me at the front door. She was wearing a sexy negligee. The only trouble was, she was coming home.

A girl phoned me and said, "Come on over. There's nobody home." I went over. Nobody was home!

A hooker once told me she had a headache.

I was making love to this girl and she started crying. I said, "Are you going to hate yourself in the morning?" She said, "No, I hate myself now."

I knew a girl so ugly that she was known as a two-bagger. That's when you put a bag over your head in case the bag over her head comes off.

My wife is such a bad cook, if we leave dental floss in the kitchen the roaches hang themselves.

I'm so ugly I stuck my head out the window, and got arrested for mooning.

The other day I came home early and a guy was jogging, naked. I asked him, "Why?" He said, "Because you came home early."

My wife's such a bad cook, the dog begs for Alka-Seltzer.

I know I'm not sexy. When I put my underwear on, I can hear the Fruit-of-the- Loom guys giggling.

George Burns

The comedy team of George Burns and Gracie Allen brought us to tears in the 60's.

George Burns and Gracie Allen Show

George Burns Roasts Jack Benny

Here are just a few on his one-liners:

First you forget names, and then you forget faces. Next you forget to pull your zipper up and finally, you forget to pull it down.

I smoke 10 to 15 cigars a day, at my age I have to hold on to something.

Everything that goes up must come down. But there comes a time when not everything that's down can come up.

A good sermon should have a good beginning and a good ending, and they should be as close together as possible.

Actually, it only takes one drink to get me loaded. Trouble is, I can't remember if it's the thirteenth or fourteenth.

When I was a boy, the Dead Sea was only sick.

Sex at age 90 is like trying to shoot pool with a rope.

Steven Wright

Steven Wright is known for his distinctively lethargic voice and slow deadpan delivery of ironic, philosophical, and sometimes nonsensical jokes. His strong Boston accent (my birthplace) just adds to it.

Here are just a few of my favorite lines from this funny guy. You can find a huge collection on the web by searching 'Steven Wright Quotes'.

If you are traveling at the speed of light in your car and turn your lights on, what happens?

I bought a humidifier and decided to buy a de-humidifier and put them in the same room and watch them fight it out.

Just before I go to get my teeth cleaned I eat a whole box of Oreo cookies.

I poured some spot remover on my dog. Now he's gone.

And here are a couple of YouTube's I think you'll love.

> Comic Relief Steven Wright Stand Up
>
> Steven Wright – Just for Laughs

"Handle each stressful situation like a dog. If you can't eat it or play with it, just pee on it and walk away."

The Beauty that Surrounds You

After losing my wife of 40 years, Jan, my life changed in so many ways. Some were expected, and some were not. One thing that I didn't expect was that I would see beauty in some of the things around me that I never gave a second thought to. And things that I thought were beautiful before the loss took on a whole new meaning. I would hear things in songs and musical pieces that I never heard before. I began to see things in pictures that I didn't remember being there before. Simple instances in nature would launch me into deep, introspective thought.

That life-changing experience taught me to see an entirely different world. The question I kept asking myself was:

"Why did I have to wait for something like this to happen before I could see all the beauty around me?"

So my advice to all of you is to focus on your world in a different way. Pretend you are a camera and look at your world using your telephoto lens, wide angle lens, cropping, portrait and landscape views etc. Look at things from as many vantage points as you can. Find the beauty in everything you see. Find things that are just downright ugly, and search for the beauty within. Find the beauty in people and things you really never cared for before. Find all the things that are beautiful about growing older. I guarantee your world will change when you do this.

You need to take advantage of this phenomenon and make it work for you. Take more walks, go to parks, notice the things around you, listen to the music and the sounds of nature, be aware of the various aromas that surround you, and experience the touch of everything you can. This will give you a great opportunity to explore the mysteries of life. You may not solve these mysteries but you'll come a lot closer to understanding them – and you'll be a better person for it.

"The darkest nights produce the brightest stars."

The Funniest Movies Ever

By now you've probably figured out that humor is a big part of my life. And it should be a big part of yours too. We all need to set aside some time for humor breaks, especially those of us who tend to take life too seriously. One way of doing this is to watch a funny movie or DVD regularly. We all have our favorites, but being the master maker of lists that I am, I have tracked my favorites through the years. And being such a nice guy, I thought I'd share them with you. Watch some of these and laugh your ever-loving butts off! Feel free to add your own favorites to this list.

Ace Ventura – Pet Detective

Airplane

Animal House

Big

Beverly Hills Cop

Blazing Saddles

Caddy Shack

Christmas Vacation

Fish Called Wanda

Happy Gilmore

The Jerk

Meet the Folkers

Monty Python and the Search for the Holy Grail

My Cousin Vinny

Naked Gun Series

Office Space

Pink Panther

Police Academy

Robin Hood – Men in Tights

There's Something About Mary

Space Balls

Stripes

Tommy Boy

Wayne's World

Young Frankenstein

"The heart has no wrinkles."

Signs That You Are Dehydrated

Water is so important to your health, and staying hydrated is so easy. All you have to do is keep that bottle of water close by, and take drinks often. Simple, huh? But it's so easy to get involved in our day to day activities and forget all about the water. So, how do you know if you are staying hydrated?

You're probably aware of the more obvious signs of dehydration: yellow urine, dry mouth, feeling thirsty. But the less-obvious signs are just as important and sometimes appear sooner, especially as you get older. The amount of water you need doesn't increase as you age, but your body's ability to conserve water is reduced and your sense of thirst weakens. So it's important to drink even if you aren't thirsty.

The importance of water can't be overstated. It makes up roughly two-thirds of our body weight and is responsible for a variety of functions, including digestion, blood flow, and temperature regulation. It's like oil to a machine. When your body is low on fluids, all systems must work harder to function properly.

So, here are a few other signs that may signal that your H2O tank is low.

You feel lightheaded or dizzy. Less water circulating in the body means less blood, too. This can lead to lower blood pressure and cause you to feel lightheaded, faint, or dizzy. One of the key signs of dehydration-related dizziness is a sudden rush of lightheadedness when you stand up too quickly.

You have bad breath. When you're dehydrated, your body secretes less fluid. You already know that means decreased urination, but it's also true for tears and saliva. Saliva is antibacterial, so if you're not producing enough, it can lead to bacteria overgrowth in your mouth. That means bad breath. It's also why so many of us experience morning breath, as saliva flow almost stops completely while we sleep. If you suddenly have dragon breath for no apparent reason, try drinking more water regularly. That alone may clear it up.

Your skin feels cold and dry. When you're approaching severe dehydration, your body starts to limit blood flow to the skin. Your body is doing what it can to conserve whatever fluid is left—even stealing water from Peter to pay Paul. The skin is the first place to be robbed of water.

You crave sweets. Dehydration can mask itself as hunger, especially in the form of sugar cravings. When you're low on fluid, your body uses glycogen (carbohydrate stored in muscle) at a faster rate, thus reducing your energy stores more rapidly. This is particularly common if you've been exercising. Your body will likely crave carbs to help replenish those glycogen stores. Before you reach for the sweets, drink some water. You might find it satisfies your craving.

You fail the pinch test. Reduced blood flow to the skin can make it feel more dough like and less elastic. If you pinch the skin on the back of your hand and it doesn't snap back as quickly as usual, it might mean you're dehydrated. Just don't expect your skin to rebound as quickly as it did in your twenties.

Listen to your body and watch for these signs of dehydration plus the more obvious ones like headache, fatigue, and yellow urine. And if you're ever concerned about hydration or experience any unusual or ongoing symptoms, talk to your doctor.

Stay hydrated by drinking at least six eight ounce glasses of water per day including a glass with every meal. Remember that fluid-filled foods such as fruits and soups and beverages such as tea and fruit juice hydrate you too. Sorry, substituting beer and wine is not a substitute.

All in all, staying hydrated looks like an easy and inexpensive way to boost your health and keep you young.

"There are two great days in a person's life – the day they are born and the day they discover why."

The 'Black Dot' Story

It's time for another story. This one has been around for a while but I try to use it frequently in thinking about my own life, and you should too. Read it through a couple of times and then play with the questions that follow.

One day a professor entered the classroom and asked his students to prepare for a surprise test. They waited anxiously at their desks for the test to begin. The professor walked around the class and handed the question papers with the text facing downwards.

Once he handed them all out, he asked his students to turn the page and begin. To everyone's surprise, there were no questions, but just a black dot in the center of the page. The professor thoroughly read through everyone's bewildered expressions and said- "I want you to write what you see there."

The perplexed students began to do what they had been asked to do.

At the end of the class, the professor took all the answer papers and started reading each one of them aloud in front of all the students. All of them with no exceptions described the black dot, trying to explain its position in the middle of the sheet, etc. After all had been read, the classroom silent, the professor began to explain:

"I am not going to grade you on this test; I just wanted to give you something to think about. No one wrote about the white part of the paper. Everyone focused on the black dot – and the same happens in our lives. This is exactly what we end to do with our lives. We have a white paper to hold onto and enjoy, but we are so busy contemplating about the dark spots that's in there. Life is a special gift and we will always have reasons to celebrate. It is changing and renewing everyday- our friends, jobs, livelihood, love, family, the miracles we see every day."

And yet we insist on focusing only on the dark spots – the health issues that are bothering us, the money that we need to have, the luxuries we don't have, complications in any relationship, problems with a family member, the disappointment with a friend and so on.

You need to realize that the dark spots are very small and only few. And yet we allow these to pollute our minds.

Take your eyes away from the black spots in your life. Enjoy each one of your blessings, each moment that life gives you.

Be happy and live a life positively!

What are the 'black spots in your life that seem to command most of your attention? Jot them down on a piece of paper.

What might you do to eliminate, or reduce these 'black spots'?

What are the 'blessings' you have in your life? Jot these down as well.

How might you focus more on these 'blessings'?

Build a list of steps you want to take in your life to begin focusing your energy on all the miracles that lie outside your life's 'black spots'.

Live life to the fullest and be happy!

"Sometimes when things are falling apart, they may actually be falling into place."

Jazz up Your Life

For as long as I can remember I have been a lover of jazz. It has to be the greatest American musical art form, period. In my days as an organizational creativity expert I would often use jazz as a metaphor for stimulating innovation in the workplace – with some great results.

Great jazz musicians are able to do three things very well. They are great technicians with their instruments and are able to perform terrific solos that bring the house down. They can also perform as a perfect team player when the band is performing as a whole. The third thing they do well (and this is a very important point) is to provide excellent background support to other soloists. So, how does this serve as a great metaphor as to how you want to live your life?

For creativity and innovation and excitement to flourish in your life you need to be a great soloist and be inventive, passionate and great at what you do. What talents and skills define you? How might you improve upon those skills? How might you make time to practice and improve these skills?

And you also need to use some of your energy and skills to support other members of your team (spouse, family, friends etc.). The act of unselfishly supporting and building on their skills creates some great camaraderie between you and your friends. How might you best use your skills to help out those you love? What are their needs, and how can you use some of your strengths to help them become great soloists as well? I think that sometimes many of us balk a bit at helping others look good because we are afraid it will make us look bad. This might be a difficult feeling to reverse but, if you can, it'll make a big difference.

And lastly, what are the best ways you can provide more subtle background support in your relationships with your friends, partners, and family? Often the best way to do this is just to be there whenever they need you. Chime in with a few of your own notes from time to time, and give them plenty of applause when appropriate. Remember, when you help others, you also help yourself.

Spontaneity, playfulness, and improvisation are other characteristics of jazz. Those in a jazz band do things from the heart because they have a high level of confidence in their individual and collective abilities. Are you making these characteristics a part of your life?

"I'll play with it first and tell you what it is later."

Miles Davis

Blueberries – The Wonder Fruit

I've often read that blueberries are good for you. But, with some further study, I have found that they are more than good for you – they are great! And, for those of you in your "mature" years, they just might be the **Wonder Fruit**. This tiny berry has been proven by physicians to aid the body with its antioxidants and nutritional properties. Here are a few reasons why the blueberry can be a good addition to a daily diet.

Combat Aging
Not only are blueberries rich in antioxidants as a whole, but they are especially rich in proanthocyandins, which have been observed to have additional anti-aging properties in several studies.

Brain Booster
According to researchers, the high level of phenols in the berry can protect the brain from degeneration, neurotoxicity, and stress.

Digestive Support
As a natural source of soluble and insoluble fiber, blueberries can help regulate the digestive system by just eating a couple of handfuls a day.

Eyesight Benefits
The anthocyanins in blueberries can protect the retina from unwanted oxygen damage. Studies also show they have been found to help protect the retina from sunlight damage.

Heart Health
A recent heart health journal showed that eating strawberries and blueberries together has a superpower tag team effect that actually decreases your risk of a heart attack by up to 33 percent.

So, get into the habit of eating fruit like this for snacks. And don't forget to have fruit smoothies often with a generous supply of blueberries. The Magic Nutri-Bullet is a great little product for making quick smoothies. I have one and love it!

"Beauty is how you feel inside, and it reflects in your eyes. It is not something physical."

Sophia Loren

What's your Vision of Your Future?

In my consulting days I spent many hours helping organizations create compelling visions of their future. I often used a quotation from hockey player Wayne Gretzky to help them along the way.

"I skate to where the puck is going to be, not to where it is."

Oftentimes we humans have a difficult time visioning a future. Our current patterns of thinking and reactive vs. creative orientation are the major blocks. So much energy goes into perpetual problem solving which may leave precious little time for creating our future. And so many of us like to stay in our comfort zones rather than risk real change.

I used a model which I called The *Journey of Discovery* and this same model may be an interesting one for you to use in creating and achieving your own vision of the future.

- Create *Viper vision*.
- Break current thinking patterns.
- Create a culture for breakthrough.
- Enhance creative thinking skills.
- Scout the future.

Viper vision creates a compelling future pull. Think about the Dodge *Viper*, a car that has no particular economic reason for being. But this car creates a vision for Dodge of what they are capable of doing, and that has made it worth its weight in gold. Try to create a "Viper vision" of your own future. What could you become if there were absolutely no constraints on your ability? Consider the following story:

The Irish writer Frank O'Connor told this story in an account of his own boyhood. He and his friends, when they were out exploring and came to an orchard wall that seemed too high to climb, would toss their hats over the wall, so that they had no choice but to follow.

What are some of the walls that seem too high for you to climb? How might you act like these boys and *throw your hat over the wall*?

What are some of the rules and assumptions (sometimes referred to as paradigms) that govern how you lead your life right now? The need to break current patterns of thinking brings about the challenging task of asking difficult questions about rules and assumptions. How might you change or shift some of these to open up more possibilities? What possibilities might exist if you break some of the rules that have governed your life up to this point?

What is the culture for change in your own situation? Does your situation allow you to risk adventuring outside your comfort zone? Are behaviors like risk taking, failing, letting go, having fun, wondering, accepting and building upon other's thinking, and being outrageous acceptable?

How might you enhance your creative thinking skills? I covered this topic fairly extensively earlier in this book and, if you really want to see some great techniques, then read one of the books in my *Creativity and Innovation Series* (another shameless plug).

And finally, you need to scout and anticipate your future. What are some things you see in the future that will help pull you forward? Describe some of the changes you may see in your future years. What do you need to do to keep up with those things that changing?

You may find this all to be a rather challenging process. But give it your best and the results may surprise you.

"Life is like riding a bicycle. To keep your balance you must keep moving."

Albert Einstein

Gardening as a Metaphor for Our Lives

I've had a passion for gardening most of my life. I was the only boy in my high school class that had a subscription to *Flower and Garden Magazine* – and I took a lot of ribbing for that. Gardening can be a wonderful metaphor for the stimulating of thoughts on how to add richness to our lives.

In a garden we:

- Plan
- Plant things (seeds, seedlings, and established plants)
- Re-arrange
- Fertilize
- Weed
- Remove bugs
- Prune
- Till soil
- Pinch back flowers
- Let wildflowers grow
- Pick flowers
- Add statuary
- Create walkways
- Protect from elements

Each one of these activities has a strong parallel with some aspects of our lives that we can influence. For example:

- How might we seed and fertilize the ideas we have to create an exciting next 50 years?
- Do we need to rearrange our priorities?
- How might we apply fertilizer to our thoughts of the future?
- How can we identify and remove the weeds that draw energy from our lives?
- What part might pruning play in the stimulation of these ideas?
- What are things we might consider pests that influence new thinking, and what can we do to combat them?
- How might we till the soil that our lives are based upon to help the creative/innovative process?
- Are there some flowers within our lives that need "pinching back" from time to time?

As you can see, the use of this metaphor allows us to pose some challenging questions while letting us carry out the conversations in a context well outside the normal thinking process.

Just think about composting. As any gardener knows, composting is a truly amazing phenomenon. How many times have you heard the cliché, *garbage in - garbage out*? In composting it's *garbage in - good stuff out*. It breaks the rules. Imagine - throw in various layers of yard and kitchen scraps, add a little *who knows what*, mix it up every now and then, give it some time and, before you know it, you've got great soil!

You may be asking what this has to do with your life. If we can create great soil out of a mixture of yard scraps and garbage, just imagine what possibilities we could achieve in our lives when we compost all our thoughts, ideas, hopes, and dreams.

Our lives are just gardens waiting to be nurtured – put those gloves on and get to work!

"The same boiling water that softens the potato hardens the egg. It's about what you're made of, not the circumstances."

Are You a Tech-Savvy Senior?

A lot of us seniors have difficulty dealing with some of the latest technology. Things have changed rapidly in the past few years, and many of us have not had the energy to keep up. You may find that all this "new stuff" is a little scary. If you have recently asked your grandchild to help you understand how to use your new Smartphone you know what I'm talking about. My daughter tells me that I am much more tech savvy than the average person of my age. I guess that's a compliment. I work pretty hard at trying to understand and work with the latest technology.

In a nutshell, here are some of the things you need to become adept at if you want to call yourself a tech savvy senior:

You need to be aware of the main sources of social media to include **Facebook, Twitter, LinkedIn, and Google +**. There are others like **Instagram, Tumbler, and Snap Chat** but they are mostly for the younger crowd. However, you may want to impress your grandchildren by becoming active on these. I personally don't feel the need here.

Start by creating your own page for each of these sites. Then join some groups, add some friends, and start some conversations. The important thing is to have fun doing this and see where it takes you.

Pinterest is another site that just beckons to seniors even though it is likely used more by the younger crowd. It's a wonderful way to express yourself via some of your major interests, and to share and gather new ideas from other users. I covered this pretty extensively in another post.

YouTube is quite simply amazing! You can find virtually anything you want on YouTube. Just go to YouTube.com and search. Want to know how to repair a left-handed wall stretcher? Just ask. Okay, that's stretching it a bit, but you get the point. Need to entertain yourself for a while? You'll find infinite options for this on YouTube.

If you want to strengthen your ability to communicate with friends and family you will need to sharpen your skills using **email, texting, Facetime, Skype** and a few other tools. Communicating with your friends and family is so easy (and usually free) these days no matter how far away they might be.

And if writing is your thing you need to gain some skills using **Microsoft Word** or an equivalent. And the ability to cut, copy, and paste is one of your greatest strengths here. Spend some time roaming around these sights and learning as much as you can. Old dogs can learn new tricks!

"You miss 100% of the shots you don't take."

Serendipity in Your Life

The word, serendipity, has a very cool ring to it. It's defined as *the occurrence and development of events by chance in a happy or beneficial way*. Many interesting new products have come from instances of **serendipity**. Lasers, televisions, cocoa cola, telephones, Velcro, the paper making process, and the first successful photographic process are all results of information that came together in serendipitous ways. And there are likely hundreds of more examples. How might you make use of this creative trigger in your own life?

You can start by staying in touch and paying more attention to what's happening around you, and spending a certain portion of your time doing things that tend to result in serendipitous thoughts. Everything is connected and everything has potential meaning for your life, so keep looking for possible connections. Great thoughts and ideas often come while wandering, wondering, day dreaming, sleeping, driving, flying, or while doing mindless tasks. So be ready for these. Mindless tasks aren't so mindless after all. I do some of my greatest thinking during these times so I make sure there is always some way of recording them (notebook, recorder etc.). These ideas tend to be fleeting - they come quick and they leave quickly, and you don't want to lose them. Most of us have Smart phones and one way of capturing these fleeting ideas is to jot them down on a "sticky note" app.

It's been said that, "*Everywhere you trip a treasure lies.*" This suggests another source of serendipity in your life. What are the things that annoy you and make you uncomfortable? Any source of pain is also a great potential source for a creative idea to reduce or eliminate that pain. Keep track of these annoyances and brainstorm things that will help avoid them.

Mistakes and accidents are frequent catalysts for new ideas. Scotch Guard, Silly Putty, laughing gas, Corn Flakes, and vulcanizing are just a few of the many examples of new products that would never have arrived if someone didn't make a mistake. Yet, we tend to think of mistakes as something to forget about rather than to learn from. Next time you make a mistake ask yourself, "What possibilities exist here and how might I take advantage of them?"

Serendipity often sprouts up while observing acts of nature. I sometimes refer to this as the **Willie Sutton logic of natural events**. Willie Sutton was a bank robber who was asked why he robbed banks. His classic answer was, "Because that's where the money is." So why not rely on nature to give us clues for new ideas? That's where the greatest ideas come from. Why not copy them? Nature is all around us and it contains some of the most powerful metaphors and triggers for new ideas. If you are having a hard time generating creative ideas to make your life more interesting the best stimulant may be as simple as taking a walk in the woods and looking for interesting connections and answers. It's also a rather enjoyable experience. Whoever said the process of generating new ideas had to be painful? As a matter of fact, having fun is a must if you really want great new idea production. New ideas come when you're able to get well outside your normal thinking domain.

At this point you may be thinking that all these things I'm suggesting are tending to force you to discover serendipity in your lives. And isn't "forced serendipity" an oxymoron? Remember the definition of serendipity refers to the 'occurrence of happy events by chance'. You can wait for these events to pop up out of nowhere – or you can engage in activities that will raise the probability of that happening. I favor the idea of venturing into areas that will create more serendipity – and maybe you should too.

"When you are tempted to give up, breakthrough is probably just around the corner."

The 'Calf Path' and the 'Roast'.

How many times have you heard the words, "That's the way it's always been done"? My guess is that you have done a lot of things in your life by making that assumption and following it. There are a couple of well known stories that illustrate this very nicely and may give us some incentive to change the way we think.

The Roast. *A young woman was preparing a roast and carefully cut off the ends. While delicious, her dinner guests wondered why she cut off the "best part." She said she did it that way because her mother always had, and her mother had taught her to prepare a roast. When she asked her mother why, the reply was that her mother, Grandma, always had as well. So they went together and asked Granny, who said, "I cut off the ends because I had a small roasting pan."*

The Calf Path. This poem written by Sam Walter Floss in the 1800's is one of the best illustrations ever on how we get stuck in our thinking, and sometimes mindlessly adhere to an established track. As you read it think of some of the ways that you may be on your own version of the calf path.

One day through the primeval wood a calf walked home as good calves should.
But made a trail all bent askew, a crooked trail as all calves do.

Since then three hundred years have fled. And I infer the calf is dead.
But still he left behind his trail. And thereby hangs my moral tale.
The trail was taken up next day by a lone dog that passed that way.

And then a wise bellwether sheep pursued the trail o'er hill and glade.
Through those old woods a path was made. And many men wound in and out and dodged and turned and bent about and uttered words of righteous wrath because 'twas such a crooked path.

But still they followed - do not laugh - the first migration of that calf.
And through this winding woody-way stalked because he wobbled when he walked.

This forest path became a lane that bent and turned and turned again. This crooked lane became a road where many a poor horse with his load toiled on beneath the burning sun, and travelled some three miles in one.

And thus a century and a half they trod the footsteps of that calf.

The years passed on in swiftness fleet. The road became a village street.
And thus, before we were aware, a city's crowded thoroughfare.

And soon the central street was this of a renowned metropolis.
And men two centuries and a half trod in the footsteps of that calf.

Each day a hundred thousand rout followed this zigzag calf about.
And o'er his crooked journey went the traffic of a continent.

A hundred thousand men were led by one calf near three centuries dead.
They followed still his crooked way, and lost one hundred years a day.
For thus such reverence is lent to well-established precedent.

Are there some situations in your life where you are putting one foot in front of the other without thinking? Take a look at some of your daily habits and ask yourself this question. Then ask yourself how you might shift your thinking and change some of these habits. Your life might just become a bit more exciting. In what ways might you create some new calf paths of your own rather than doing things because "that's the way it's always been done"?

"Sometimes it's the smallest decisions that can change your life forever."

Cleaning Out the Garages of Your Life

Have you ever spent a day cleaning out your garage or cellar and then found that it really made you feel good? I sure have. Well why not apply this theory to your life. We tend to collect a lot of stuff through the years, and much of it tends to just get stored away, never to be seen again. Or sometimes it just becomes a source of something more to worry about. The older we get, the more important it becomes to simplify our lives.

Get rid of anything that isn't **useful, beautiful, or joyful** to you. There is stuff all around us, stuff in our heads, and, for those who spend a lot of time in the digital world, stuff in our computer files. A good metaphor for this whole process is the reconfiguration and defragmentation of computer drives. Every time I do this I feel better for some reason. Sometimes we just need to defragment our minds.

Here are some of the things that you should simplify.

Simplify Your Schedule. Here is an interesting and simple way of looking at how to really clean up your schedule.

- Make a list of things that make you happy.
- Make a list of things you do every day.
- Compare these lists.
- Adjust accordingly

How many things are taking up your time that don't either make you happy or add excitement and beauty to your life? Make a list of things you HAVE to do and a list of things that you WANT to do. What are some of the things on the HAVE to list that you can sacrifice to give you more time for your WANTS? Can you plan your day so that it includes special time periods to assure that you are doing some of the things you really want to do? For example, among other things, I love to read, write, and listen to music. So I set aside certain times during the day to do these. Some of the things you love can be done simultaneously (like listening to music while writing), so work on building your multi-tasking skills.

Simplify Your Expectations – Shoot From the 'Golds'. Sometimes, when we are feeling stressed out, it may be because we are expecting too much of ourselves. You may expect to be perfect at everything. You may have a need to be better than your friends and associates. You may have set your goals much too high. If your expectations are too complex and out of reach your inability to achieve them may make you very unhappy. Take a serious look at your expectations and reposition and resize them so they are challenging, but achievable. And, if you find you just have too many expectations, eliminate a few that really aren't that important.

So what do I mean when I say, 'shoot from the 'golds'? If you are a golfer this will make a lot of sense to you. Most courses have multiple tee sites (blue, white, gold, and red) based up on the golfer's ability, gender, or age. I am by no means a great golfer but felt that I should always shoot from the 'whites'. That is until a friend told me that I would enjoy the game much more if I played from the 'golds'. He said I've earned it because of my age – and he was dead right. My game is so much more enjoyable now.

Downsize Your Stuff. George Carlin did a wonderful skit which was all about "stuff". Check it out on YouTube if you can before you read any further. I remember back when I had a growing family and decided to get one of those storage sites so that I could make more space in my home for more stuff. When my kids all left home I decided to close this, and ended up throwing out almost everything I had stored – for years!

It feels great when you downsize. Pick a certain spot and begin cleaning. Attics, cellars, garages, and closets are great starting points. Throw out or sell anything that you haven't used in a while. You may discover a lot of things which you've long ago forgotten about. Spend a little time dwelling on the nice memories some of these bring to you. Some of those rediscoveries may still add value to your life – you don't have to toss everything. And you will likely find that your family may love a lot of those things you no longer need. Why not distribute some of your stuff to your family and friends? And there is always the possibility of selling them on EBay. This could be a pretty good source of some extra *pin money.*

Cast Aside Your Negative Thoughts. Negative thoughts have the power to block you from true happiness. Through the years, a lot of us develop negative thoughts about a number of things. There may be certain people you don't like. Perhaps you have developed a strong bias or prejudice about certain people, politics, religions, lifestyles, practices, etc. I am the first to admit that I once had some negative thoughts about some of these things. But I have tried my best to eliminate these, and I think I have succeeded. And I feel much better because of this.

One method I used to suggest to my clients was to write all of your negative thoughts on some toilet paper, and then flush them. Sounds crazy – but it works!

So here is what you need to do. Take a careful look at each of these areas for downsizing and simplifying your life. Have fun and enjoy the process. After you have succeeded in downsizing, focus on maintaining a simpler, less complicated life, and make sure you don't slip back to where you were before.

For those in their golden years it is important to make sure that those loved ones who you will leave behind are not left dangling. Obviously having a will is of utmost importance. And I'm going to go out on the limb a bit and suggest that a large majority of you either don't have a will, or have one that is outdated. A lot of folks move to friendlier climates when they retire without realizing that a will from one state may not be applicable in another state. Without a will your family might be subjected to some vultures that are waiting to get a piece of your estate – and I'm sure you wouldn't want to have that happen. If you have shied away from doing this because of the perceived cost there are a number of websites and some very inexpensive software available. One I have found to be very easy and friendly is **Will Maker**. You may also want to try **LegalZoom.com**.

Writing about this reminds me of a story I heard recently about an elderly gentleman who had a hearing problem. He finally decided to get some hearing aids and was pleasantly surprised that he could now hear all the conversations that went on within his family. His doctor asked him how his family felt about how he could finally hear their conversations.

His comment was, "I haven't told them I can hear them yet, and I've changed my will 3 times already".

Start cleaning right now!

"Enjoy the little things in life because one day you will look back and realize that they were the big things."

What You Can Learn from Bumper Stickers

Ah, the world of bumper stickers. They have always fascinated me. Bumper stickers are a way of making statements and putting them out for the whole world around you to see. I see everything as a learning experience, and bumper stickers are no exception. Here are a few of these from those I have collected through the years. In what ways do they trigger some new thoughts about your own situation?

- Lottery: A tax on people who are bad at math.
- Consciousness: The annoying time between naps.
- Be nice to your kids. They'll be choosing your nursing home.
- We all live downwind.
- If the people lead then eventually the leaders will follow.
- Sometimes I wake up Grumpy. Sometimes I let her/him sleep.
- Change is inevitable, except in vending machines.
- Your kid may be an honor student but you're still an idiot.
- Why be normal?
- Subvert the dominant paradigm.
- Minds are like parachutes, they only function when open.
- My karma ran over your dogma.
- Everything I know is a result of my ignorance.
- Compost happens.
- They are not hot flashes – they are power surges.
- Enjoy life- this is not a dress rehearsal.
- A bad day fishing is still better than a good day at work.
- Alcohol and calculus don't mix. Never drink and derive.
- In dog years, I'm dead.
- Gravity – It's not just a good idea. It's the law.
- If at first you don't succeed, skydiving isn't for you.
- Old age comes at a bad time.
- The more you complain the longer God makes you live.
- If you can read this I can hit my brakes and sue you.
- If we are what we eat, I'm cheap, fast, and easy.
- Fake it until you make it.
- Just undo it.
- We have enough youth. How about a fountain of smart?
- Question authority.
- Politicians and diapers need to be changed often for the same reason.
- Enjoy life. This is not a dress rehearsal.
- Forget world peace. Visualize using your turn signal.
- New York – where politicians make our license plates.

"Aging is not lost youth, but a new stage of opportunity and growth."

Have a Whine and Jeez Party

At one point in my life I was, among other things, what I might call a 'Creative Process Consultant'. In a nutshell, my job was to help various teams to change the way they think so they could develop breakthrough possibilities. I used a variety of home grown techniques to begin the process of changing their thinking. In many cases these teams came with a lot of cranial baggage, and I would often begin by trying to get this out of their systems.

I invented a technique I called, *'The Whine and Jeez Party'*. One of my many observations about teams in general was that they tended to complain a lot – and sometimes whine a lot. My thought was that, if I could create a process that allowed them to unload all the issues that bothered them, it would be a good start for them to begin some breakthrough thinking. And guess what – it really worked!

So what does this have to do with how to stay young? We all have issues that build up through the years that bother us and impede our ability to move on. These could be personal issues or ones that deal with our relationships with friends and family or, perhaps, just things that bug you. So why not schedule a 'Whine and Jeez Party' of your own? You could start with your own personal party where you just whine to yourself about all the things that bother you. And then you could schedule a party with a selected group of family or friends to whine about all the things that collectively bother you.

The important thing is to make this a fun experience – try not to take it too seriously. Whine about all the things that bug you – big or small. And it may help to have some real wine and cheese there too. If you have a group of people, begin by having everyone walk around and whine about something to others in the group. Try to have them use the "whiniest' voice possible - that adds to the fun. And when the whining is done have a conversation about what just happened, and how everyone feels about it. How did this change your thinking about how you want to move on?

There's a good chance you will find that this activity will help you clean out some of the cobwebs in your mind and allow you to think clearer about your future. It's amazing how the simple act of verbalizing your concerns can help to clear them up. You may even want to have a monthly 'Whine and Jeez Party'.

*"A bird doesn't sing because it has an answer.
It sings because it has a song."*

Have Your Own Humor Room

I don't know about you but I just can't imagine life without humor. Back in my days as an engineer and creative thinking expert for Kodak I designed and built what was arguably the first corporate humor room ever. I was intensely interested in the effect of humor in the workplace and did a lot of pioneering work on how to eliminate the oxymoron of 'fun work'. Accessing the humor in your life has so many benefits, and I think I've covered them very well in other parts of this book. So why can't we create 'humor rooms' in our own lives?

'Humor rooms' are places to get charged, recharged, excited, stimulated, humored, challenged, unstressed, turned on, and transformed. They can come in all sorts of shapes and sizes. A 'humor room' could actually be a room in your domain that houses lots of humor material. Or perhaps you'd like to scatter humorous material all about your home so that everywhere you went would have the capacity to make you laugh. Your entire home would then be your 'humor room'

Your 'humor room' might consist of keeping some humorous photos on your computer or having several Pinterest boards that focus on various humor sources (funny cartoons or quotations, YouTube's of your favorite comedians, etc.).

Perhaps your 'humor room' would be the placement of some slightly weird and funny pictures, furniture, or objects around your home.

Here are a few items you may want to make a part of your 'humor room':

- Posters of your favorite comedians
- Some of you favorite humorous quotations
- A few gag gifts (a rubber chicken is a must)
- A few humorous videos like Jeff Foxworthy, Monty Python, and the Carol Burnet show, etc.
- A library of funny books to include my books of course, Dave Barry, Far Side, and any others that make you laugh
- A marginally weird clock, lamp, or other accessory
- Toys and stuff for juggling (balls, scarves, hamburgers, chain saws etc.)
- Anything else that makes you laugh

Have fun with this and I'd love to hear some stories about how you put this to use. Send me a note at lindsaycollier@comcast.net with your story. I'll be in my own 'Humor Room'.

"Laughter is the fireworks of the soul."

Senior Discounts

There is one great advantage to being a senior - there are a lot of discounts available to you. You can find this information easily on the web but I thought I'd share it here, especially for those of you who may not be web browsers. This information is all subject to change but this will give you a good starting point. There are also a lot of discounts for those of you who are Veterans as well. Don't be afraid to take advantage of these – you've earned them. And don't be afraid to ask any vendor not on the list if they too have discounts.

Go to theseniorlist.com for a more detailed list of specific discounts. Here is a partial list of various categories that offer senior discounts:

- Restaurants. There is a long list of these but, if your favorite is not on the list, ask and 'maybe you shall receive'.
- Hotels. Probably every hotel has a senior discount but other options might be cheaper (AAA, Choice Privileges etc.).
- Movies. Most movie houses offer discounts, mostly for daytime use.
- National Parks. If you visit these often you should look into buying a Golden Pass which will give you free access as a senior.
- Amusement parks. Most amusement parks love seniors since they are often dragging along a bunch of grandkids.
- Cruises.
- Stores. Many stores have what they call, *Senior Days*, with some very good discounts.
- Airlines.
- Car rentals and public transport.
- Medicines. There are a lot of options for seniors in this area to discover.
- Home Refinancing. HARP, veteran's loans, and reverse mortgages are something you may want to explore if interested in refinancing your home.

As a veteran you are entitled to a number of benefits. Go to militarybenefits.info for more detailed information. Both Home Depot and Lowes offer a 10% discount to veterans which can come in real handy. Go to their service desks with your DD214 and they will set it up for you. And don't be afraid to ask any vendor if they have veteran's discounts. They will probably say yes and, if they say no, they should be quite embarrassed. You've earned it big time! Florida (and perhaps some other states as well) has an option to have your veteran status on your license which comes in handy for identification purposes. Check your local licensing bureau for information.

"I'm not getting old. I'm just becoming a classic."

Develop Your Own Job Title

Job titles have always fascinated me. As a former engineer I had a rather nondescript title up till the time that I decided I would make up on my own which was based on the particular passion I was following. From time to time my passions shifted around a bit so I would change my title accordingly. I still think that having a title that expresses your current passion is a great idea.

What are the things that currently excite you and really turn you on? What are some of the things at which you excel? How would your friends describe you? Or, better still, how would you like them to describe you? Brainstorm some possible titles that best describe these thoughts. Select one for starters and make that your current title. A title that makes you and others laugh is a pretty good start. You may even want to go as far as making a few business cards if you can. Here are a few starters for you, but don't let that keep you from coming up with your own original.

- Chief Gadfly
- Purveyor of Outrageously Interesting Ideas
- Glutton for Funishment
- Rattler of Bushes/Ruffler of Feathers
- Keeper of Pit Bulls for Mouth Foaming Creativity
- Purveyor of Feet in the Backside
- Slayer of Sacred Cows
- Mistress of Chaos
- Royal Stardust Keeper
- Yah-Butt Blaster
- Supreme Allied Commander
- Mind Mine Sweeper
- Catcher of All That Hits Fans
- Wild Thing
- Sand Box Monitor
- Heel Nipper
- Happily Ever After Maker
- Empress of the Universe
- Resident Disturber of the Peace
- Raging Inexorable Thunder-Lizard Evangelist
- Wild Thing
- All That Is Powerful and Wise

- Big Kahuna
- Muckety Muck
- Duchess of Danger
- Troublemaker
- Director of Fun
- Master of Madness
- Vibe Evolver
- Pride Piper of Creativity
- Idea Gooser
- Chief Creatologist
- Myth Debunker
- Resident Dreamer
- Seer, Inspirer, and Spark Plug
- Wizard of Wonder
- Hope Builder
- Super Simplifier
- Cerebral Proctologist
- Chief Imagination Officer
- Insight Manager
- Human Being
- Director of Everything
- Squeezer of Thinking Juices
- Manager of Mischief

"You miss 100% of the shots you don't take."

Find Your *Thinkorarium*

Several years ago my son and I were on our annual upstate New York fall leaf gawking trip. We happened on a place called the Glen Curtiss Museum in Hammondsport, NY, a very picturesque town on the southern edge of Keuka Lake in the Finger Lakes region. What a great find! Glen Curtiss was one America's most inventive minds, and here's a museum full of his inventions. Since we were both Mechanical Engineers we had to stop and spend a few hours there. Curtiss lived on a hill overlooking Keuka Lake and had a cupola mounted on his house that contained a room he called his *Thinkorarium*. That cupola is the centerpiece of the museum. This is where he went to do his best thinking. Everyone should have one of these. For the longest time I couldn't get the idea of *a thinkorarium* out of my mind.

A *thinkorarium* doesn't even have to be a place. It could be anything you do that tends to bring out your best and most creative thinking. Einstein liked to become whatever his problem was. 'Let me ride on that light wave for a while and see what it's like'. Bucky Fuller liked to create words (like *tensegrety*) that created a *thinkorarium* in his mind. You may find your best *thinkorarium* is simply letting your mind wander. You just need to find that special place, and go there often.

If there is a special room in your home that gives a little boost to your thinking, then add a few things that will help trigger your creativity. This could be pictures, objects, music, weird furniture or accessories, etc. Perhaps there's a special place in your yard that allows your mind to wander. Some people (including me) do some of their best thinking while driving. Make your car your *thinkorarium* and keep a small recorder handy to save your thoughts. Often new ideas come while sleeping. Have you ever woken because of an interesting thought that popped into your head? Keep a small notebook handy, because there's a good chance that idea might be long gone when you wake up.

The internet is one of the greatest sources of ideas. There is an infinite amount of interesting information at your fingertips, and this might be where your own personal best thinking takes place. So, take some time each day to visit your *thinkorarium* and begin capturing your creative thoughts. Don't forget to have your notebook or journal handy.

"Even if you are on the right track you'll get run over if you just sit there."

Joe Santoro

Revisiting the Abilene Paradox

At one point in my career I was quite involved in team building. I often used a story that was quite popular at the time that well illustrated the problem of 'group think'. This story was developed by Jerry Harvey of George Washington University, in 1974. The parable goes like this:

A husband, wife, and her parents are sitting cozily in the porch of their house in Coleman, Texas. The day is hot, and they're busy sipping lemonade, whiling away their time. There is a suggestion by the father-in-law to drive about 53 miles to Abilene, to eat at a cafeteria. The other three are apprehensive, yet agree to it, deciding to go with the flow, rather than opposing it. They end up going to Abilene, in a non-air conditioned car, in the scorching heat, and come back home, having a not-so-great lunch. On their way back, they moan and complain that the decision was wrong, and that they did not want to go in the first place, but stuck to it, since they did not want to go against the will of others. The person who had suggested the idea (father-in-law) also states that he simply suggested it because he thought the others might be bored. Eventually, they end up wondering why they wasted their resources on something which none of them wanted to indulge in.

Interesting, isn't it? This situation has been named *'driving to Abilene'*, since many times, we end up taking a decision because of a lack of courage to express our real thoughts, and end up having to accept an unwanted decision, which leads to the road to 'Abilene'. After reading this story, I'm sure there will be many real-life examples that will come to mind.

Are there times when you have just gone with the flow and later regretted that decision?

Are there any unwanted situations in your life today that are a result of "*driving to Abilene*"?

Have you ever been in a situation where you ended up fuming and fretting and wished you had spoken up?

I'm reminded of a song of the past called '*Silence is Golden*'. Don't you believe this one bit. Next time you are tempted to go along with something that you don't want, speak up. Bring up some good alternatives if you can, or just refuse. You've earned it. Just say to them, "Abilene is not on my bucket list'.

"You're never too old to do goofy things."

Beware of Falling

Often when I meet with my doctor or nurse practitioner they ask a series of questions about my general health. One of the questions they now ask (I assume because of my age) is whether I have fallen lately. And, I must admit that a number of my friends have been experiencing more falls. Risk of falling does increase as we age, but there are a lot of things we can do to lessen this risk.

There are three categories of fall risks:

- Heath - based risks. This includes things like balance problems, weakness, chronic illnesses, vision problems, and medication side-effects. They are specific to an individual person.
- Environmental risks. These are things like home hazards (e.g. loose throw rugs), outside hazards (e.g. icy sidewalks), or risky footwear (e.g. high heels). This category can also include improper use of a walker, cane, or other assistive device.
- Triggers. These are the sudden or occasional events that cause a challenge to balance or strength. They can be things like a strong dog pulling on a leash, or even health-related events like a moment of low blood sugar (hypoglycemia) in a person with diabetes.

Perhaps the best advice should come straight from your doctor's mouth. The next time he or she asks you if you have experienced falling, be honest. My first thought when asked this was that I would be embarrassed if I said yes. Don't feel that way! Falls are the leading cause of both fatal and nonfatal injuries for people over 65! They can result in hip fractures, broken bones, and head injuries.

At the very minimum, here are a few things you can do to minimize the risk of falling:

- Have an annual checkup of your vision. This is important for a number of reasons, one of which is to assure that vision problems are not contributing to your risk of falling.
- Make a safety assessment of your home and surroundings to minimize anything that might cause a fall.
- Exercise regularly and include exercises that focus on balance.
- If you experience dizziness seek your doctor's advice to find the root cause.

Enjoy staying upright!

"Do something today that your future self will thank you for."

Nows, Wows, and Holy Cows

In one of my first books, **Organizational Mental Floss**, I include dozens of techniques I have used in my career as an expert in creative thinking. This particular technique may help your provide some interesting possibilities for your future. It's a fast and fun way to take your thinking up a few notches concerning the possibilities of adding some zest to your life.

The first step is to jot down a few statements that describe your life today. These are the NOWS. Think of your current situation including (but not limited to) your:

- Possessions
- Relationships
- Hobbies and Interests
- Beliefs
- Finances
- Desires

For each of these develop a sub list of WOWS. In what ways might you take each of these up a notch? For example, if you are focusing in on your interests and one of them is listening to music, one of your WOWS might be to take up an instrument. You're probably thinking that it's too late to do something like this. As a matter of fact, at this point there may be a strong tendency to think of all the reasons that these WOWS can't happen. Try your best not to let that happen! You can make anything happen if you really put your mind to it. I have known several people who have taken up an instrument late in life and have done very well.

And now for the HOLY COWS. Select a few items from your WOW list and begin to really stretch your thinking. This is the time for some **mental bungee jumping** which I mentioned in an earlier article Have some fun with this and don't be afraid to get a little crazy. Using the previous example of taking up an instrument, some HOLY COWS might be to start or join a band, write your own compositions, make a CD, or try out for America's Got Talent. The higher your goal, the more exciting your endeavor will be.

Based on this process, summarize a few scenarios of the things you want to aim for in your future.

"The past is a place of reference, not residence."

The Starfish Story

Here's another story that has been around for a while. I used this years ago when training people in the art of creative thinking. It's still as meaningful as it was back then.

A young man is walking along the ocean and sees a beach on which thousands and thousands of starfish have washed ashore. Further along he sees an old man, walking slowly and stooping often, picking up one starfish after another and tossing each one gently into the ocean.

"Why are you throwing starfish into the ocean?" he asks.

"Because the sun is up and the tide is going out

And, if I don't throw them further in they will die."

"But, old man, don't you realize there are miles and miles of beach and starfish all along it?

You can't possibly save them all, you can't even save one-tenth of them. In fact, even if you work all day, your efforts won't make any difference at all."

The old man listened calmly and then bent down to pick up another starfish and threw it into the sea. "It made a difference to that one."

Are there some things in your life you would like to change, but have hesitated because it seemed like such an awesome task, and you didn't know where to start? I believe that is true of many of the goals we would like to achieve. The best way to achieve success may be to begin by taking a small step. Small steps will help us to move forward to our goals, and also give us energy and momentum to keep on rolling.

So next time you feel that reaching a certain goal in your life is impossible, throw out a starfish, and start moving forward.

"You can't steal second base if you keep your foot on first base."

Dealing With Loss in Your Life

Several years ago I lost my wife of 40 years, Jan, to ovarian cancer. The following day a huge rainbow surrounded my home in Rochester, New York which inspired me to write *Surviving the Loss of Your Loved One, Jan's Rainbow*. As we grow older the fact is that we will tend to experience the loss of family and friends. And, if you have ever lost a pet dog or cat, you know how difficult that can be as well. I have experienced a lot of loss in my own lifetime and this has taught me a great deal as to how to deal with it. So here are a few words of advice to you.

Turn each loss into a learning experience. What can I learn from the experience of losing someone I truly cared about? Set aside some time for deep thinking and meditating and time to learn as much as you can about loss, dying, and grieving. Find a place or an activity that allows you to do this such as a peaceful spot or a walk in the park. Read some books on loss to help you better understand the process of grieving and the meaning of death.

Losing someone you love can literally rock your world, and erode your self-esteem and confidence. It can give you a beaten down feeling like you've just been through a wringer. But as Bernie Segal once said;

> *"If God puts you through a wringer, it's because you are worth laundering."*

Turning the whole process into a learning experience can help you in a big way to regain your confidence and optimism.

Reframe your thinking. Reframing can be a very powerful way to create new, more positive ways to think about your problems. It involves looking at various aspects of your situation and creating more positive ways of thinking of them. Here are a few examples.

'How will I be able to live without him?' becomes 'How wonderful it was to have this person in my life.'

'She won't be with me anymore' becomes 'I can keep her in my heart

forever.' 'Dwelling on their sickness' becomes 'Remembering their wellness.'

'Thinking of her pain' becomes 'Remembering her laughter and her smile.'

Use as a stepping stone to turn yourself into a better, more caring person.
After losing Jan my daughter told me that losing her Mom made her realize that she wanted to experience her life to the fullest. Part of this is doing whatever you can to help others who are experiencing loss. My book on how to survive loss has given comfort and

hope to so many people, and this in turn has helped me in my own recovery. When you help someone out you always help yourself as well.

- In what ways might the loss of your loved one give higher meaning to your life?
- How might you become a better person based on the experience of your loss?
- In what ways might you help others who are also grieving?

To the extent you can, play an active role in helping the family of those you have lost by staying in touch and providing helpful advice and understanding.

Stay connected with others who have experienced similar loss. After my loss I joined a bereavement group and, to this day, I feel it saved my life. After losing someone you love, one of your biggest needs is to have someone to talk to. And the best people are those who are going through the same thing you are experiencing. Do not shy away from joining a bereavement group if your situation calls for it. There are many of these available through churches, senior groups, and hospice organizations, and they are extremely helpful.

- What are some possible groups that you can join in your area? (Hospice organizations, churches, etc.)
- Are there some old friends or associates that have experienced a similar loss that you should contact?

Dealing with the loss of loved ones in your life will be one of your biggest challenges. Always aim at trying to give this challenge a positive spin no matter how difficult this seems. There is always light at the end of the tunnel.

"Loss makes artists of all of us as we weave new patterns in the fabric of our lives."

Greta W. Crosby

Senior Scams

Remember the days when we could trust just about everyone? It looks like those days are over, and there's a plethora of scams these days, many of them targeting seniors. The National Council on Aging (ncoa.org) has a very nice website to provide help to seniors in a number of areas, including senior scams. Technology today has made it rather easy for scammers since the internet gives them a huge playground. And seniors often make handy targets for them.

The key thing to keep in mind is that, when you see an email or get a phone call that's suspicious, **do not respond**. Take appropriate action whether it be deleting, hanging up, or reporting it to the authorities. And never agree to give to charities that solicit by phone – simply tell them you do not accept these calls.

Following are a few of the scams to watch out for:

Grandparent Scams. If you ever get a call from someone pretending to be a grandchild or relation who is in trouble and needs money, do not fall for it. If it seems to be real (very unlikely) ask a lot of key questions to establish proof. They will probably hang up.

Email/phishing scams. These are very common and very easy to fall prey to. One thing to always keep in mind is to never give anyone your social security number or other important numbers. The usual message tells you that there has been some suspect activity on one of your accounts (normal a bank) and that you need to verify or update your information. **Banks do not send messages via email.** Delete this message and contact the bank if you want to take it further. There is also a common scam that involves calls from the IRS telling you that you are in trouble. Stay as clear from them as you can!

Investment schemes. Seniors who are looking to maximize their savings might tend to fall for a variety of schemes (pyramids, princes that want to share their inheritance etc). The key is to always work with financial consultant that you trust.

Fraudulent or useless anti-aging products. There are a plethora of products out there that promise to make you look 20 years younger. Few of them will do what they say, so make sure to carefully study the reviews before trying them.

Funeral and cemetery schemes. Those who are bereaving loss are more susceptible to fraud. If you find yourself in that position beware of anyone who makes claims on the deceased, and also beware of funeral homes that try to sell you unneeded extras.

Counterfeit prescription drugs. Drugs play an important part in the lives of many seniors, but counterfeit drugs are quite common. The danger here is that you may be wasting money, but you may also be putting yourself in danger with these drugs.

Medicare and health insurance scams. There is probably nothing more important in the lives of seniors than having a good health care program. There is also nothing that can get as confusing as figuring out what is best for you. Unfortunately, this creates a good breeding ground for scammers. Make sure you are dealing with a legitimate agent for all your health insurance needs.

Homeowner re-financing offers. Seniors who own their homes are often barraged with offers to refinance at low rates. There are legitimate offers in this area but you need to be aware of those that do not deliver what they promise.

This is a quick overview of some common senior scams. There is a pile of information on these on the internet if you would like more detail. Be careful and stay safe.

"Reset. Refocus. Restart. Readjust. As many times as you need to."

Myths about Growing Old

Growing older is inevitable, but growing old is not. There's a lot you can do to make your second fifty years your best fifty. The first step is to debunk all those myths about growing old. Remember, YOU ARE WHAT YOU THINK. And, if you can think young, you have a good chance of growing young. Age is just a number!

A common stereotype of a senior is an older person who has a memory attention of a couple of minutes, spends their day gawking out the window, is cranky, is either frail or overweight, and walks like a duck. Okay, maybe that's a slight exaggeration. But, let's face it; some people may feel that way. Truth is there a lot of seniors who are getting better with age – like fine wine. Let's take a look at a few myths about aging.

Your brain turns to mush. As we age, we do lose certain aspects of our brain function such as memory of specific events and details. But the good news is that we have accumulated a wealth of information and insights that a younger person lacks. Complex decision making requires experience and wisdom which means that seniors are quite capable of some really great thinking.

The same goes for emotional intelligence and verbal ability. And what might seem like slower mental response time may actually signal the overstuffed memory files in your brain. One thing I have noticed is that my ability to multi-task has lessened. If that is the case with you, simply don't try to do as many things at once.

All that said, your brain might turn to mush if you don't use it and exercise it. Many of the articles in this book have addressed this and I suggest you make sure to have a daily program in play to keep your brain healthy. Travel, try new things, socialize with an array of people, and do a variety of brain challenging exercises daily.

You can't learn new things. The old saying that "you can't teach old dog new tricks" is not true. It just sometimes takes a little longer. As you age, you can and should learn new things. The fact that our brains are full of 'old things' can often get in the way of this learning. Much of our learning may have to be preceded by some' unlearning'. And never let the observation that your grandchildren are smarter than you get in the way

Intimacy becomes a thing of the past. Some studies show that intimacy and sexual satisfaction is higher when you are young (no surprise here), lower in your middle years, and then increases in senior years (surprise!) . Don't give up on your chance for intimacy just because of your age. Think of yourself as getting better and don't be afraid to try new forms of intimacy. We all need intimacy in our lives.

Your muscle will turn to mush. It's true that you lose a certain amount of muscle mass with each decade of aging. But you CAN get this back through proper exercise. You may have to give up your dream of becoming 'Mr. or Mrs. Universe', but that's okay.

Resistance exercise is important because it helps to build up mass. You can do this using weights, resistance bands, or bodyweight, and also through everyday tasks such as gardening. Another advantage to maintaining muscle mass is that, the stronger you are, the less likely you are to fall. And, if you do fall, you'll have some padding to cushion the blow.

Your appetite goes away. Actually, there is a certain amount of truth to this. I can't eat the portions that used to be normal for me – and I think that's a good thing. As we get older, our stomachs empty a little more slowly so we tend to get fuller more quickly. Our bodies lose muscle and we exercise less, so we require fewer calories. And our taste buds become less sensitive. The important thing is to make sure your weight stays in the healthy range. If your eating habits are changing and causing weight gain or loss, it's time to do something about it.

You become a grim, cranky person. Getting older doesn't have to turn you into a total crank. It all starts with not being so serious about life. Loosen up, laugh a lot, smile at everything and everyone, and try your best to be the ultimate optimist – no matter what's going on in your life.

So let's all get over these myths and begin growing young!

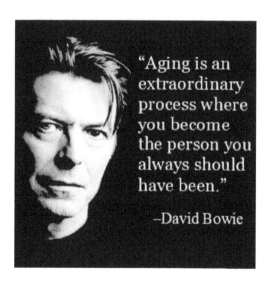

"Aging is an extraordinary process where you become the person you always should have been."

–David Bowie

Getting Your Ducks in a Row - Rebooting, and De-fragmenting Your Life

I'm on my computer a lot and seem to experience a number of slowdowns, seizures, and crashes. Fortunately none have been too serious, and I always seem to be able to solve the problem by restarting, rebooting, and defragmenting. It sometimes reminds me of my own brain. As a writer I sometimes have what is often called 'writer's block'. I sit down at my computer ready to write some good stuff – and nothing happens. There are some days when you have the same experience with other activities as well.

Perhaps it's time to reboot and defragment. I'm not an expert with computers but I think of defragmentation as a form of 'getting your ducks in a row'. This reminds me of a quotation I recently came across.

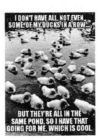

Life seems to be a series of 'ups' and 'downs'. That's pretty normal and should not give you cause to worry. If you are riding on a long 'up', then good for you. But if you are experiencing a long 'down', it may be time for a reboot. A very long one may suggest depression in which case you should seek help. Here are some questions that may help you along the way in your rebooting process.

Where am I now?

Where do I want to be?

In what ways might I get there?

What are my ducks and how can I put them in a row?

Rebooting and defragmentation processes on your computer are always followed by shutting down and restarting. Try to relax and shut down your brain for a while and then restart with a new perspective. Hopefully this will result in a nice long 'up'.

"Not all storms come to disrupt your life; some come to clear a path."

Challenging Your Senses

We have five senses; sight, hearing, taste, smell, and touch. Each of these senses provides us with a particular view of the world around us. We are usually quite satisfied with using each of the senses for their assigned purpose. But, what if you were able to challenge these senses to do something a little different? At one point in my life as a creative thinking consultant I would use this technique to get groups to ratchet up their thinking. And it worked! Why not give it a try?

As an example, we usually use our senses of vision and smell to examine a rose. What does a rose sound like, taste like, feel like? Your favorite song sounds wonderful. But how does it smell, taste, feel, and look like? Listen to the smell of a delightful perfume. What might you hear? See the sound of some instruments in an orchestra. What does the sound of a flute look like to you? What does the sound of the bass drum look like? How does red feel to you? How does the blue sky feel to your touch? How does gray flannel taste to you?

At this point you may think I'm nuts – and maybe you are right. But sometimes you need to try some crazy things to get on a new thinking path.

Take a few minutes and try to:

- See what you can hear.
- Hear what you can touch
- Feel what you can taste.
- Smell what you can see.
- Taste what you can smell

Now use this technique to create some new thoughts about the life ahead of you. What possibilities arise from looking at this using all five senses? What does your future sound like, look like, feel like, smell like, and taste like? Have some fun with this and see what happens.

"Nothing you wear is more important than your smile."

When I Buy the Farm

Here's a final thought. So many of my posts and blurbs on how to grow young come from a perspective of 'living forever'. I'm an eternal optimist and like to think of life this way. But, let's face it; sooner or later we will all 'buy the farm'. What would you want to tell your family and friends before this happened? Don't wait till it's too late. Think about the loved ones you will be leaving behind and put yourself in their shoes. What do you think they would like to hear you say, and how might you add comfort to what they will be going through?

There are a surprising number of folks that do not have wills or, if they do have them, have not kept them up to date. Wills get out of date with time. If you have moved to another state, your will may not even be valid anymore. Without a will, your family may have a difficult time during probation, and your state might end up with a big chunk of the proceeds. So, get that will done. If finances limit what you can spend on this, then look for available software or apps which may work just fine.

Here are a few things you may want to include in your message:

A personal message to those you love. What would you say if you had just one hour left with them? Tell them how wonderful it was to have them in your life. Let them know some of the wishes you have for their future. What are some things that you have never told them but wish you had? Remember, the idea of this is to give them comfort as they grieve your loss. Write from your heart and try not to be deadly serious. Use of some humor in your message will make it even more comforting.

Your eulogy and epitaphs. What would you like to be said about you if there is a funeral? What would you like to see on your gravestone?

Your specific desires for burial and funeral arrangements. Do you want to be buried, cremated, buried at sea, frozen al la Ted Williams etc? If cremated, what do you want done with the ashes? These are all questions they will have on their minds, and a little advice from you might help.

Who gets your stuff. If you have a will, this will dictate the disposal of your major assets. But what about all the stuff you have collected through the years? Your photos, memorabilia, treasures, collections, tools, vehicles, furniture, home goods etc. will all need a home. Why not give some guidance to those you are leaving behind on who should get these items?

Putting this all in writing will give you great peace of mind, and those you leave behind will be very thankful.

"I never lose. Either I win or I learn."

Parting Words and an Extra Bonus

I have had a blast putting this book together and hope you have enjoyed it. I also hope you were able to grab onto a lot of ideas that will add zest to your life. I invite you to follow my Growing Young blog at growingyoungsite.wordpress.com. Please tell your friends about the book and the blog. And I would love to have you share any thoughts or ideas with me via my email, lindsaycollier@comcast.net. **I just love receiving messages from my readers!**

I always like to leave all my readers with a smile on their face and some laughter in their soul, so here are some of my favorite senior jokes. Jokes about aging are pretty popular among my contemporaries. After all, there's not much we can do about it other than joke about it. So here are some of the best jokes I've ever seen on the topic of growing old (which I preferred calling *growing young*).

Senior Jokes and Funny Stuff

Aging Gracefully

I changed my car horn to gunshot sounds. People move out of the way much faster now!

I didn't make it to the gym today (that makes five years in a row).

I changed calling the bathroom "the John" and renamed it "the Jim" (I feel better saying I went to "the Jim")!

Last year I joined a support group for procrastinators. We haven't met yet...

I don't need anger management. I need people to stop irritating me!

When I was a child, Nap Time was a punishment... Now, as a grown up, it feels like a small vacation....

My people skills are just fine. It's my tolerance of idiots that needs working on.

If God wanted me to touch my toes, he would have put them on my knees.

The kids text me "plz"... is shorter than "please". So, I text back "no" (because it's shorter than "yes").

I'm going to retire and live off of my savings. Not sure what I'll do the second week.

Even duct tape can't fix stupid... *but it can muffle the sound*!

Of course I talk to myself... sometimes I need expert advice.

Elders Texting

An elderly couple had just learned how to send text messages on their mobile phones. The wife was a romantic type and the husband was more of a no-nonsense guy.

One afternoon the wife went out to meet a friend for coffee.
She decided to send her husband a romantic text message and she wrote:

"If you are sleeping, send me your dreams.

If you are laughing, send me your smile.

If you are eating, send me a bite.

If you are drinking, send me a sip.

If you are crying, send me your tears.

I love you."

The husband texted back to her:

"I'm on the toilet. Please advise."

The Importance of Walking and Exercise

Walking can add minutes to your life. This enables you at 85 years old to spend an additional 5 months in a nursing home at $7000 per month.

My grandpa started walking five miles a day when he was 60. Now he's 97 years old and we don't know where he is.

I like long walks, especially when they are taken by people who annoy me.

The only reason I would take up walking is so that I could hear heavy breathing again.

I have to walk early in the morning, before my brain figures out what I'm doing..

I joined a health club last year, spent about 400 bucks. Haven't lost a pound. Apparently you have to go there.

Every time I hear the dirty word 'exercise', I wash my mouth out with chocolate.

The advantage of exercising every day is so when you die, they'll say, 'Well, she looks good doesn't she.'

If you are going to try cross-country skiing, start with a small country.

I know I got a lot of exercise the last few years, just getting over the hill.

We all get heavier as we get older, because there's a lot more information in our heads. That's my story and I'm sticking to it.

Every time I start thinking too much about how I look, I just find a Happy Hour and by the time I leave, I look just fine.

A Letter from a Nice Old Lady

God bless you for the beautiful radio I won at your recent senior citizens luncheon. I am 84 years old and live at the Springer Home for the Aged. All of my family has passed away. I am all alone now and it's nice to know that someone is thinking of me. God bless you for your kindness to an old forgotten lady. My roommate is 95 and has always had her own radio, but before I received one, she would never let me listen to hers, even when she was napping.

The other day her radio fell off the night stand and broke into a lot of pieces. It was awful and she was in tears. Her distress over the broken radio touched me and I knew this was God's way of answering my prayers. She asked if she could listen to mine, and I told her to kiss my ass.

Thank you for that opportunity.

Grandson's Prayer

Dear God, please send clothes for all those poor ladies on Grandpa's computer. Amen.

Mike and Yvonne

Mike and Yvonne were 85 years old and had been married for sixty years. Though they were far from rich, they managed to get by because they carefully watched their pennies. Though not young, they were both in very good health, largely due to Yvonne's insistence on healthy foods and exercise for the last decade.

One day, their good health didn't help when they went on a vacation and their plane crashed, sending them off to Heaven. They reached the pearly gates, and St. Peter escorted them inside. He took them to a beautiful mansion, furnished in gold and fine silks, with a fully stocked kitchen and a waterfall in the master bath. A maid could be seen hanging their favorite clothes in the closet. They gasped in astonishment when he said, 'Welcome to Heaven. This will be your home now.'

Mike asked Peter how much all this was going to cost. 'Why, nothing,' Peter replied, remember, this is your reward in Heaven.' Mike looked out the window and right there he saw a championship golf course, finer and more beautiful than any ever built on Earth. 'What are the greens fees?' grumbled Mike. 'This is heaven,' St. Peter replied. 'You can play for free, every day.'

Next they went to the clubhouse and saw the lavish buffet lunch. 'Don't even ask,' said St. Peter to Mike. This is Heaven, it is all free for you to enjoy.' Mike looked around and nervously asked Yvonne 'Well, where are the low fat and low cholesterol foods and the decaffeinated tea?'

'That's the best part,' St. Peter replied. 'You can eat and drink as much as you like and you will never get fat or sick. This is Heaven!'

'No gym to work out at?' said Mike. 'Not unless you want to,' was the answer.

'No testing my sugar or blood pressure or...' 'Never again'

Mike glared at Yvonne and said, 'You and your dam Bran Flakes. We could have been here ten years ago!

The Old Guy and the Trooper

A Florida senior citizen drove his brand new Corvette convertible out of the dealership.

Taking off down the road, he pushed it to 80 mph, enjoying the wind blowing through what little hair he had left. "Amazing," he thought as he flew down I-95, pushing the pedal even more.

Looking in his rear view mirror, he saw a Florida State Trooper, blue lights flashing and siren blaring. He floored it to 100 mph, then 110, then 120. Suddenly he thought, "What am I doing? I'm too old for this!" and pulled over to await the trooper's arrival.

Pulling in behind him, the trooper got out of his vehicle and walked up to the Corvette. He looked at his watch, and then said, "Sir, my shift ends in 30 minutes. Today is Friday. If you can give me a new reason for speeding – a reason I've never before heard – I'll let you go.."

The old gentleman paused then said, "Three years ago, my wife ran off with a Florida State Trooper. I thought you were bringing her back."

"Have a good day, Sir," replied the trooper.

Jacob and Mary

Jacob, age 92, and Mary, age 89, living in Fort Myers, are all excited About their decision to get married. They go for a stroll to discuss The wedding, and on the way they pass a drugstore. Jacob suggests they go in. Jacob addresses the man behind the counter.

"Are you the owner?" The pharmacist answers, "Yes."

"We're about to get married. Do you sell heart medication?" Pharmacist: "Of course we do."

"How about medicine for circulation?" Pharmacist: "All kinds."

"Medicine for rheumatism?" Pharmacist: "Definitely."

"How about suppositories and medicine for impotence?" Pharmacist: "You bet!"

"Medicine for memory problems, arthritis and Alzheimer's?" Pharmacist: "Yes, a large variety. The works."

"What about vitamins, sleeping pills, Geritol, antidotes for Parkinson's disease?" Pharmacist: "Absolutely."

"Everything for heartburn and indigestion?" Pharmacist: "We sure do."

"You sell wheelchairs and walkers and canes?" Pharmacist: "All speeds and sizes."

"Adult diapers?" Pharmacist: "Sure."

"We'd like to use this store as our Bridal Registry."

60th Anniversary

He was a widower and she a widow. They had known each other for a number of years being high school classmates and having attended class reunions in the past without fail. This 60th anniversary of their class, the widower and the widow made a foursome with two other singles. They had a wonderful evening, their spirits high. The widower threw admiring glances across the table; the widow smiled coyly back at him. Finally, he found the courage to ask her, "Will you marry me?" After about six seconds of careful consideration, she answered, "Yes,..... yes I will!"

The evening ended on a happy note for the widower. But the next morning he was troubled. Did she say "Yes" or did she say "No?" He couldn't remember. Try as he would, he just could not recall. He went over the conversation of the previous evening, but his mind was blank. He remembered asking the question but for the life of him he could not recall her response. With fear and trepidation he picked up the phone and called her.

First, he explained that he couldn't remember as well as he used to. Then he reviewed the past evening. As he gained a little more courage he then inquired of her. "When I asked if you would marry me, did you say "Yes" or did you say "No?"

"Why you silly man, I said 'Yes. Yes I will.' And I meant it with all my heart."
The widower was delighted. He felt his heart skip a beat.

Then she continued. "And I am so glad you called because I couldn't remember who asked me!"

Elderly Couple On a Cruise

An elderly couple was on a cruise and it was really stormy. They were standing on the back of the boat watching the moon, when a wave came up and washed the old woman overboard.

They searched for days and couldn't find her, so the captain sent the old man back to shore with the promise that he would notify him as soon as they found something.

Three weeks went by and finally the old man got a fax from the boat. It read: "Sir, sorry to inform you, we found your wife dead at the bottom of the ocean. We hauled her up to the deck and attached to her butt was an oyster and in it was a pearl worth $50,000. Please advise.

"The old man faxed back: "Send me the pearl and re-bait the trap."

Maude and Claude

Maude and Claude, both 91, lived in The Villages, in Florida. They met at the singles club meeting and discovered over time that they enjoyed each other's company. After several weeks of meeting for coffee, Claude asked Maude out for dinner and, much to his delight, she accepted. They had a lovely evening. They dined at the most romantic restaurant in town. Despite his age, they ended up at his place for an after-dinner drink.

Things continued along a natural course and age being no inhibitor, Maude soon joined Claude for a most enjoyable roll in the hay. As they were basking in the glow of the magic moments they'd shared, each was lost for a time in their own thoughts.....

Claude was thinking:

'If I'd known she was a virgin, I'd have been gentler.'

Maude was thinking:

'If I'd known he could still do it, I'd have taken off my pantyhose.'

Doctor's Exam

After an examination, the doctor said to his elderly patient: 'You appear to be in good health. Do you have any medical concerns you would like to ask me about?'

'In fact, I do.' said the old man. "After my wife and I have sex, I'm usually cold and chilly; and then, after I have sex with her the second time, I'm usually hot and sweaty."

When the doctor examined his elderly wife a short time later he said, 'Everything appears to be fine. Are there any medical concerns that you would like to discuss with me?' The lady replied that she had no questions or concerns. The doctor then said to her, 'Your husband mentioned an unusual problem. He claimed that he was usually cold and chilly after having sex with you the first time; and then hot and sweaty after the second time. Do you have any idea about why?'

"Oh, that crazy old bastard" she replied. 'That's because the first time is usually in January, and the second time is in August.

Grandfather

I want to die peacefully in my sleep like my grandfather.
Not screaming in terror like his passengers.

Old Man And The Beaver

An 86-year-old man went to his doctor for his quarterly check-up. The doctor asked him how he was feeling, and the 86-year-old said, 'Things are great and I've never felt better.' I now have a 20 year-old bride who is pregnant with my child. "So what do you think about that Doc?"

The doctor considered his question for a minute and then began to tell a story. "I have an older friend, much like you, who is an avid hunter and never misses a season." One day he was setting off to go hunting. In a bit of a hurry, he accidentally picked up his walking
cane instead of his gun."

"As he neared a lake, he came across a very large male beaver sitting at the water's edge. He realized he'd left his gun at home and so he couldn't shoot the magnificent creature. Out of habit he raised his cane, aimed it at the animal as if it were his favorite hunting rifle and went 'bang, bang'.

"Miraculously, two shots rang out and the beaver fell over dead. Now, what do you think of that?" asked the doctor.

The 86-year-old said, "Logic would strongly suggest that somebody else pumped a couple of rounds into that beaver."

The doctor replied, "My point exactly."

A Few Thoughts About Growing Old

My memory's not as sharp as it used to be. Also, my memory's not as sharp as it used to be

It's scary when you start making the same noises as your coffee maker.

I've sure gotten old! I've had two bypass surgeries, a hip replacement, new knees, fought prostate cancer and diabetes. I'm half blind, can't hear anything quieter than a jet engine,
take 40 different medications that make me dizzy, winded, and subject to blackouts. Have bouts with dementia. Have poor circulation; hardly feel my hands and feet anymore.
Can't remember if I'm 85 or 92. Have lost all my friends. But, thank God, I still have my driver's license

The New Hearing Aid

A man was telling his neighbor, "I just bought a new hearing aid. It cost me four thousand dollars, but it's state of the art."

"Really," answered the neighbor. "What kind is it?"

"Twelve thirty."

Morris

Morris, an 82 year-old man went to the Doctor to get a physical. A few days later the doctor saw Morris walking down the street with a gorgeous young lady on his arm. A couple of days later the doctor spoke to the man and said, "You're really doing great, aren't you?" Morris replied, "Just doing what you said, Doc: 'Get a hot mamma and be cheerful.' "

The Doctor said, "I didn't say that. I said you got a heart murmur. Be careful."

The Freeway

As a senior citizen was driving down the freeway, his car phone rang. Answering, he heard his wife's voice urgently warning him, "Herman, I just heard on the news that there's a car going the wrong way on 280 Interstate. Please be careful!"

It's not just one car," said Herman. "It's hundreds of them!"

Endearing Terms

An elderly gent was invited to his old friends' home for dinner one evening. He was impressed by the way his buddy preceded every request to his wife with endearing terms-- Honey, My Love, Darling, Sweetheart, Pumpkin, etc. The couple had been married almost 70 years and, clearly, they were still very much in love.

While the wife was in the kitchen, the man leaned over and said to his host, "I think it's wonderful that, after all these years, you still call your wife those loving pet names."

The old man hung his head. "I have to tell you the truth," he said, "I forgot her name about 10 years ago.

Senior Sex

On hearing that her elderly grandfather had just passed away, Katie went straight to her grandparent's house to visit her 95- year old grandmother and comfort her. When she asked how her grandfather had died, her grandmother replied, "He had a heart attack while we were making love on Sunday morning."

Horrified, Katie told her grandmother that 2 people nearly 100 years old having sex would surely be asking for trouble. "Oh no, my dear, "replied granny. "Many years ago, realizing our advanced age, we figured out the best time to do it was when the church bells would start to ring. It was just the right rhythm. Nice and slow and even. Nothing too strenuous, simply in on the Ding and out on the Dong."

She paused, wiped away a tear and then continued, "and if that damned ice cream truck hadn't come along, he'd still be alive today!!!

Old Man from Idaho

An old man lived alone in Idaho. He wanted to spade his potato garden, but it was very hard work. His only son, Bubba, who used to help him, was in prison. The old man wrote a letter to his son and described his predicament.

Dear Bubba,
I am feeling pretty bad because it looks like I won't be able to plant my potato garden this year. I'm just getting too old to be digging up a garden plot. If you were here, all my troubles would be over. I know you would dig the plot for me. Love Dad

A few days later he received a letter from his son.

Dear Dad
For heaven's sake, dad, don't dig up that garden, that's where I Buried the BODIES. Love Bubba

The next morning, F.B.I. agents and local police showed up and dug up the entire area without finding any bodies. They apologized to the old man and left. That same day the old man received another letter from his son.

Dear Dad
Go ahead and plant the potatoes now. It's the best I could do under the circumstances Love Bubba.

Viagra

They finally released the ingredients of Viagra:

3% Vitamin E
2% Aspirin
2% Ibuprofen
1% Vitamin C
20% Spray Starch
67% Fix-A-Flat

The Vacuum Cleaner Salesman

A little old lady answered a knock on the door one day, only to be confronted by a well-dressed young man carrying a vacuum cleaner. "Good morning," said the young man. "If I could take a couple of minutes of your time, I would like to demonstrate the very latest in high-powered vacuum cleaners."

Bug off!" said the old lady. "I haven't got any money" and she proceeded to close the door. Quick as a flash, the young man wedged his foot in the door and pushed it wide open. Don't be too hasty!" he said. "Not until you have at least seen my demonstration." And with that, he emptied a bucket of horse poop all over her hallway carpet.

"If this vacuum cleaner does not remove all traces of this horse poop from your carpet, Madam, I will personally eat the remainder." "Well," she said, "I hope you've got a freaking good appetite, because the electricity was cut off this morning."

Elderly Man in Phoenix

An elderly man in Phoenix calls his son in New York and says, "I hate to ruin your day, but I have to tell you that your mother and I are divorcing, forty-five years of misery is enough."

"Pop, what are you talking about?" the son screams.

"We can't stand the sight of each other any longer, "the old man says. " We're sick of each other, and I'm sick of talking about this, so you call your sister in Chicago and tell her," and hangs up.

Frantic, the son calls his sister, who explodes on the phone. "Like heck they are getting divorced," she shouts, "I'll take care of this." She calls Phoenix immediately, and screams at the old man, "You are not getting divorced. Don't do a single thing until I get there. I'm calling my brother back, and we'll both be there tomorrow. Until then, don't do a thing, DO YOU HEAR ME?" and hangs up.

The old man hangs up the phone and turns to his wife. "Okay," he says. "They're coming for Thanksgiving and paying their own way"!

90 - Year Old Grandfather

My friend John went to visit his 90 - year old grandfather in a very secluded, rural area of Saskatchewan. After spending a great evening chatting the night away, the next morning John's grandfather prepared breakfast of bacon, eggs and toast. However, John noticed a film like substance on his plate, and questioned his grandfather asking,

'Are these plates clean?'

His grandfather replied, 'They're as clean as cold water can get them. Just you go ahead and finish your meal, Sonny!'

For lunch the old man made hamburgers. Again, John was concerned about the plates, as his appeared to have tiny specks around the edge that looked like dried egg and asked,

'Are you sure these plates are clean?'

Without looking up the old man said, 'I told you before, Sonny, those dishes are as clean as cold water can get them. Now don't you fret, I don't want to hear another word about it!'

Later that afternoon, John was on his way to a nearby town and as he was leaving, his grandfather's dog started to growl, and wouldn't let him pass. John yelled and said, 'Grandfather, your dog won't let me get to my car'. Without diverting his attention from the football game he was watching on TV, the old man shouted!

'Coldwater, go lay down now, yah hear me!'

Sixty Five Year Old Mother

With all the new technology today regarding fertility, a 65 year old woman was able to give birth. When she was discharged from the hospital and back home her friend visited her.

"May I see the baby", she asked. "Not now", said the mother. "Let's have a cup of coffee and chat for a while".

Thirty minutes passed and she asked, "Can I see the baby now?" "No.", said the mother. After several more minutes she asked again and the mother said, "No, not yet".

Growing quite impatient, she said, "Well, when can I see the baby?"

"When he cries", said the mother.

"When he cries? Why do I have to wait until he cries?" she demanded.

"Because I forgot where I put him, O.K?"

The Fairy Godmother

A married couple in their early 60s was celebrating their 40th wedding anniversary in a quiet, romantic little restaurant.

Suddenly, a tiny yet beautiful fairy appeared on their table. She said, 'For being such an exemplary married couple and for loving each other for all this time, I will grant you each a wish.'

The wife answered, 'Oh. I want to travel around the world with my darling husband.' The fairy waved her magic wand and - poof! - two tickets for the Queen Mary appeared in her hands.

The husband thought for a moment: 'Well, this is all very romantic, but an opportunity like this will never come again. I'm sorry my love, but my wish is to have a wife 30 years younger than me.'

The wife, and the fairy were deeply disappointed, but a wish is a wish.

So the fairy waved her magic wand and - poof!-the husband became 92 years old.

Old is When:

Your sweetie says, 'Let's go upstairs and make love,' and you answer, 'Pick one; I can't do both!'

Your friends compliment you on your new alligator shoes and you're barefoot.

A sexy babe or hunk catches your fancy and your pacemaker opens the garage door.

Going braless pulls all the wrinkles out of your face.

You don't care where your spouse goes, just as long as you don't have to go along.

You are cautioned to slow down by the doctor instead of by the police.

'Getting a little action' means you don't need to take any fiber today.

'Getting lucky' means you find your car in the parking lot.

An 'all-nighter' means not getting up to use the bathroom.

You get the same sensation from a rocking chair that you once got from a roller coaster.

When you fall down you wonder what else you can do while you're down there.

Everything either dries up or leaks.

There is a snap, crackle, and pop in the morning, and no Rice Crispi's.

You're at the beauty shop for two hours, and that was just for an estimate.

All the names in your address book end in M.D.

You start making the same noises as your coffee maker.

Half the stuff in your shopping cart says, "Fast Relief".

You and your teeth don't sleep together.

Happy hour is a nap.

Your idea of weight lifting is standing up.

It takes longer to rest than it did to get tired.

You sink your teeth into a steak, and they stay there.

You wonder how you could be over the hill when you can't even remember being on top of it.

The Perks of Getting Older

In a hostage situation, you are likely to be released first.

Things you buy won't wear out.

Your investment in health insurance is finally paying off.

Your joints are more accurate meteorologists than the national weather service.

You can sing along with elevator music.

Your supply of brain cells is finally down to a manageable level.

Your secrets are safe with your friends because they can't remember them.

Aging Artists

Some of the artists of the 60's are now in their golden years. So they are revising the titles of their hits to accommodate the baby boomers.

They include:

Bobby Darin – Splish, Splash, I Was Havin' a Flash.

Hermin's Hermits – Mrs. Brown, You've Got a Lovely Walker. Ringo Starr – I Get By With a Little Help from My Depends. The Bee Gees – How Can You Mend a Broken Hip?

Roberta Flack – The First Time I Ever Forgot your Face.

Johnny Nash – I Can't See Clearly Now.

Paul Simon – Fifty Ways to Lose Your Liver.

The Commodores – Once, Twice, Three Times to the Bathroom.

Marvin Gaye – Heard it Through the Grape Nuts.

Procol Harem – A Whiter Shade of Hair.

Leo Sayer – You Make Me Feel Like Napping.

The Temptations – Papa's Got a Kidney Stone.

Abba – Denture Queen.

Tony Orlando – Knock 3 Times On the Ceiling If You Hear Me Fall.

Helen Reddy – I Am Women, Hear Me Snore.

Leslie Gore – It's My Procedure, and I'll Cry If I Want To.

Willie Nelson – On the Commode Again.

Other Books by Lindsay Collier

Amazon.com/author/lindsaycollier

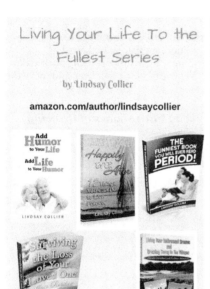

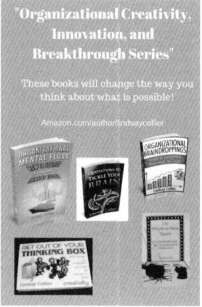

One Last Thing

If you found this book helpful and believe it is worth sharing, would you take a few seconds to let your friends know about it? If it turns out to make a difference in their lives, they will be forever grateful to you, as I will.

In addition, if you have a few moments now to leave a short review on the Amazon product page, please, please do. Something that just takes a few moments will help me out today and for years to come. Your support really does make a difference, and I read all the reviews personally so I can get your feedback and make the book even better

All my best to you, and thank you so much for reading *Fifty Shades of Growing Old*.

Made in the USA
Coppell, TX
14 November 2021